Contemporary Issues in Fetal and Neonatal Medicine

3

Ethical Issues at the Outset of Life

Contemporary Issues in Fetal and Neonatal Medicine

3

Ethical Issues at the Outset of Life

EDITED BY
WILLIAM B. WEIL, JR., M.D.
MARTIN BENJAMIN, Ph.D.

Blackwell Scientific Publications

BOSTON   OXFORD   LONDON

EDINBURGH   PALO ALTO   MELBOURNE

Blackwell Scientific Publications
Editorial Offices
52 Beacon Street, Boston,
 Massachusetts 02108, USA
Osney Mead, Oxford OX20EL, England
8 John Street, London, WC1N 2 ES,
 England
23 Ainslie Place, Edinburgh, EH3 6AJ,
 Scotland
107 Barry Street, Carlton, Victoria 3053,
 Australia
667 Lytton Avenue, Palo Alto,
 California 94301, USA

Distributors
USA
 Year Book Medical Publishers, Inc.
 35 East Wacker Drive
 Chicago, Illinois 60601
Canada
 Blackwell Mosby Book Distributors
 120 Melford Drive
 Scarborough, Ontario M1B 2X4
Australia
 Blackwell Scientific Publications,
 Pty., Ltd.
 107 Barry Street
 Carlton, Victoria, 3053
Outside North America and Australia
 Blackwell Scientific Publications, Ltd.
 Osney Mead
 Oxford OX2 0EL
 England

Typeset by TC Systems, Inc.
Printed and bound by Edwards Brothers, Inc.

Library of Congress Cataloging in
Publication Data

Ethical issues at the outset of life.

 (Contemporary issues in fetal
and neonatal medicine ; 3)
 Includes bibliographies and index.
 1. Perinatology—Moral and ethical
aspects. I. Weil, William B.
II. Benjamin, Martin. III. Series.
[DNLM: 1. Ethics, Medical.
2. Perinatology. W1 C0769MQP
v.3 / WQ 210 E84]
RG600.E84 1987   174'.2   87-15796
ISBN 0-86542-046-7

To Andrew D. Hunt, founding Dean of the College of Human Medicine at Michigan State University, whose appreciation of interdisciplinary work in medicine and the humanities fostered the generative environment in which this book was conceived.

Contents

Contributors

JOHN D. ARRAS, Ph.D.
Department of Epidemiology and Social Medicine
Albert Einstein College of Medicine
Yeshiva University
Bronx, New York

WILLIAM G. BARTHOLOME, M.D.
Associate Professor
Pediatrics and the History and Philosophy of Medicine
College of Health Sciences and Hospital
University of Kansas
Kansas City, Kansas

MARTIN BENJAMIN, Ph.D.
Department of Philosophy
Michigan State University
East Lansing, Michigan

ALAN R. FLEISCHMAN, M.D.
Director of Neonatology
Albert Einstein College of Medicine
Yeshiva University
Bronx, New York

JOHN C. FLETCHER, Ph.D.
Chief, Bioethics Program
Warren G. Magnuson Clinical Center
National Institutes of Health
Bethesda, Maryland

ROBERT A. HAHN, Ph.D., M.P.H.
E.I.S. Officer
Epidemiology Research Branch
Division of Sexually Transmitted Diseases
Centers for Disease Control
Atlanta, Georgia
Note: Dr. Hahn's chapter is not a publication of the Centers for Disease Control.

RUTH MACKLIN, Ph.D.
  Professor of Bioethics
  Albert Einstein College of Medicine
  Yeshiva University
  Bronx, New York

THOMAS H. MURRAY, Ph.D.
  Professor of Medical Humanities
  Institute of Medical Humanities
  University of Texas Medical Branch
  Galveston, Texas

PETER SINGER, Ph.D.
  Director
  Centre for Human Bioethics
  Monash University
  Clayton, Victoria
  Australia

CARSON STRONG, Ph.D.
  Associate Professor
  Department of Human Values and Ethics
  College of Medicine
  University of Tennessee
  Memphis, Tennessee

WILLIAM B. WEIL, JR., M.D.
  Professor
  Department of Pediatrics/Human Development
  Michigan State University
  East Lansing, Michigan.

Preface

Advances in perinatal medicine have created a number of bewildering ethical issues. New reproductive technologies, such as *in vitro* fertilization and embryo placement, raise difficult questions about the nature of the family and the moral status of the embryo. New information about the relationship between fetal development and maternal behavior, as well as the development of certain forms of fetal therapy and surgery, create additional conflicts between the interests of the fetus and those of the pregnant woman. And advances in neonatal intensive care generate troubling dilemmas about when, if ever, life-sustaining treatment should be withheld from a seriously ill newborn.

The difficulties are compounded when they arise in a pluralistic society. A person's views about these matters are not fully determined by abstract, impersonal reason. The values governing our convictions about sexuality, family, birth, and death are also related to sentiment and personal, cultural, and historical circumstance. Where these differ, as they usually do in avowedly pluralistic societies, people's positions on issues in perinatal ethics will also differ, and the power of abstract, impersonal reason to resolve the issues to everyone's satisfaction will be correspondingly limited. Yet the issues have public as well as private dimensions that cannot be ignored. Although our convictions about sexuality, family, birth, and death are rooted in differing world views and ways of life, a society and its health care institutions must have certain more or less singular laws and policies about such matters. To leave all decision-making to individual conscience where individual consciences differ and yet physicians, nurses, and patients of differing beliefs must work closely together in pursuing a uniform course of action is to invite chaos. Thus an important, yet vexedly difficult, problem in a pluralistic society is to determine exactly what its laws and policies should be when various members have radically divergent and rationally irreconcilable convictions about the ethics of such issues as *in vitro* fertilization, abortion, and withholding aggressive treatment from seriously ill newborns. Law and public policy in other contested areas often involve a certain degree of compromise. Is it likely, or even possible, that parties to disputes in perinatal ethics might also agree to certain forms of compromise with regard to questions of law and public policy?

A principal aim of this book is to show the connections between all of these matters—to provide, as it were, a rough geography of the field of perinatal ethics. Issues having to do with the creation of life, pregnancy, newborn intensive care, and public policy are usually discussed separately. By presenting them together we hope to display a number of illuminating connections and to contribute to the development of more comprehensive and coherent resolutions. A related aim is to provide introductions to specific topics and areas that will convey a general understanding of relevant issues, concepts, and arguments, as well as the point of view of a distinguished contributor to ongoing debates and discussion.

Chapter 1 presents an overview of the entire range of issues in perinatal ethics. Like the book as a whole, it has a developmental structure that begins with issues that arise during the preimplantation period and then proceeds to the intrauterine and postnatal periods. The concluding section addresses questions of public policy in a pluralistic society as they apply to all three periods.

Chapter 2, by Peter Singer, Director of the Centre for Human Bioethics at Monash University in Australia, is on the creation of human embryos. Singer defends what he calls the "simple case" of *in vitro* fertilization in which a married infertile couple use an egg taken from the wife and sperm taken from the husband, and all embryos created are inserted into the womb of the wife. After addressing a number of standard objections to the "simple case," Singer turns to a discussion of other cases and the question of the moral status of the embryo. In the next chapter, John C. Fletcher, Chief of the Bioethics Program at the National Institutes of Health, examines various issues raised by genetic assessment. He provides detailed, up-to-date introductions to the major ethical questions in prenatal diagnosis, genetic counseling, and genetic screening, and he makes a number of thoughtful recommendations for dealing with them.

Chapters 4 and 5 address issues that arise during pregnancy. Chapter 4, by William G. Bartholome, Associate Professor of Pediatrics and the History and Philosophy of Medicine at the University of Kansas, discusses the termination of pregnancy from the perspective of the physician. The standpoint of the physician is, according to Bartholome, neglected in current debates and needs to be more fully appreciated. The physician's perspective, he suggests, is inseparable from that of the pregnant woman and the relationship between them. In Chapter 5 Alan R. Fleischman, Director of Neonatology at the Albert Einstein College of Medicine, and Ruth Macklin, Professor of Bioethics at Albert Einstein, examine the ethical considerations and potential conflicts that arise from various types of fetal therapy. Fleischman and Macklin carefully identify the principal ethical issues and approach them with a sensitive and sophisticated emphasis on the consequences of various possible alternatives.

In Chapter 6 philosopher John Arras of the Department of Epidemiology and Social Medicine of the Albert Einstein College of Medicine discusses the uses and abuses of the notion of the "quality of life" in neonatal ethics. Arras's careful analysis tries to point out the limits of quality of life reasoning as well as the extent to which it is inescapable. The following chapter, by Carson Strong of the Program on Human Values and Ethics at the University of Tennessee, focuses on the extent to which parents should be allowed to participate in treatment decisions for their seriously ill newborns. The main difficulties with such participation in the past, Strong suggests, have been rooted in poor interaction between physicians and parents. He concludes with a number of suggestions for improving this relationship in the neonatal context.

The final chapters turn to questions of public policy raised by ethical issues in perinatal ethics. Medical anthropologist Robert A. Hahn, currently with the Centers for Disease Control, suggests in Chapter 8 that different ethnic groups in the United States (Navajo, Chinese, lower class blacks, and middle-class whites) and one group of professionals (American obstetricians) have importantly different and occasionally conflicting ethical perspectives with regard to perinatal matters. As a result, Hahn suggests, the prospects for a "transcultural perinatal ethics" that would readily resolve all of our differences are, at best, quite dim. Then, in Chapter 9 Thomas H. Murray, Professor of Medical Humanities at the University of Texas Medical Branch at Galveston, addresses the more normative question of how a pluralistic society ought to formulate public policy on matters as central and bitterly contested as those in perinatal ethics. It is one thing, Murray maintains, to have what one regards as a well-grounded moral conviction on an issue in perinatal ethics and quite another to believe that it, and it alone, ought to become public policy in a pluralistic society. The aim of his chapter, Murray writes, "is [to] give some sense of the kinds of values that come into play at the level of social policy, and to stress the independent importance of them over and above the values determining the morality of the particular practice, be it abortion, IVF [in vitro fertilization], or decision making for seriously ill newborns."

As a work in philosophical medical ethics, this book does not pretend to dispense authoritative answers or definitive solutions to the questions raised. The authors are all active participants in an ongoing, complex, societal "conversation" about ethical issues at the outset of life. They would agree that the worth of a particular position in perinatal ethics is a function of the cogency of the underlying reasons and not of the identity, eminence, or credentials of the person who states it. Their aim in contributing these original essays, then, is not to terminate the public conversation, but rather to enlarge and deepen it. Well-grounded, stable solutions or adjudications to most issues in perinatal ethics will require the thoughtful, informed participation of large numbers of scholars, health care professionals, citizen-patients, and policy-makers. It is the hope of all who have contributed to this book that it will enable the reader to follow the ongoing discussions and debates more readily and to contribute to them more effectively.

I

Introduction and Overview

1

Ethical Issues at the
Outset of Life

MARTIN BENJAMIN and WILLIAM B. WEIL

It used to be much simpler: sexual intercourse, pregnancy, and birth, followed by the usual joys and sorrows of parenthood. But advances in medicine and technology together with rapidly changing social conditions and expectations have now turned what was for centuries a more or less routine part of the life cycle into a source of personal confusion and social debate.

Prior to pregnancy, new ways of creating life and new techniques of genetic assessment appear to many to threaten the nature and meaning of human relationships and reproduction. During pregnancy, the combination of a more thorough understanding of fetal development and new possibilities for fetal surgery, on the one hand, and deep social division about the permissibility of abortion and the rights of women, on the other, generate apparent conflicts between the interests of the fetus and those of the pregnant woman. After birth, the uncertain prognosis for many recipients of newborn intensive care raises difficult questions about whether certain lives are of such low quality that they should not be sustained and about who, if anyone, is qualified to make such decisions. Finally, all of these questions raise difficult issues not only for the affected patients, parents, and health care professionals, but for society at large. How can a pluralistic society develop coherent policies on such matters while respecting the plausible, yet conflicting and rationally irreconcilable, viewpoints of many of its members?

In what follows we provide an overview of each of these problem areas and show connections between them. This will provide background for the more detailed essays in the remainder of the book. Our discussion, like the book as a whole, will have a developmental structure. We begin with ethical issues that arise during the preimplantation period and then turn to the intrauterine and postnatal periods. We conclude by raising questions of public policy as they apply to all three periods.

Preimplantation

Efforts to overcome infertility have resulted in a number of new ways of creating human life. These in turn have raised a number of ethical issues

3

for prospective parents, physicians, and society. Less exotic, but no less problematic, are a number of questions that arise out of advances in human genetics. Like new techniques for overcoming infertility, genetic assessment, counseling, and screening solve or ameliorate some problems while creating or aggravating others.

Making Babies

Approximately 15 percent of couples wanting to have children are infertile, with the causes divided evenly between the partners. In response, modern medicine has developed a number of remedies ranging from artificial insemination to *in vitro* fertilization and embryo placement. Yet nearly every technical advance seems to leave in its wake possibilities and implications that range far beyond the more immediate concern of correcting or compensating for the infertility of a husband and wife.

Although artificial insemination with a husband's sperm (AIH) raises difficulties only for those whose objections to interference with nature would count equally well against nearly any medical intervention, artificial insemination with sperm from a donor (AID) is more problematic. Should the donor be screened for genetic or other medical problems? Should the donor remain anonymous? If so, what if it is later important in the course of the child's medical treatment to know something about the medical history of his or her biological parents? And must AID be restricted to married couples? What if a single woman or a lesbian couple want to have a natural child without having a sexual relationship with a man?

Matters become even more complicated when we turn to techniques for overcoming female infertility. Since the birth of the first "test tube" baby in 1978, over 4,000 children have been created through *in vitro* fertilization (IVF) and embryo placement (EP). In the standard case ova from a wife are fertilized in a petri dish with sperm from her husband and then placed in the uterus. Skilled practitioners achieve pregnancy in 20 to 30 percent of their attempts. For others the success rates are lower. Thus far the incidence of chromosomal and genetic defects following IVF appears to be no greater than that following ordinary reproduction. In the standard case, then, IVF and EP seem to be more complex technically, but no more problematic ethically, than AIH. Yet new ethical questions arise when IVF and EP include the freezing and storing of embryos and when they involve parties other than a husband and wife.

Since the chances of pregnancy resulting from any instance of IVF and EP are about 1 in 5 (with some clinics doing better and some worse), a number of attempts at EP must usually take place before implantation is achieved. To reduce the number of laparoscopies needed for egg retrieval, techniques have been developed to allow for the removal of a number of ova at one time. All are then fertilized. A few of the resulting embryos are placed in the uterus with the hope that one will implant, while the remainder are frozen and then stored for subsequent attempts if they should prove necessary. Problems arise, however, about the status of such embryos if they are not later needed or wanted by this couple for EP. May they be destroyed? May they be used in research? Such questions raise deep and difficult questions about the nature and value of human life. For if one believes that life begins at conception, that it is always wrong to take innocent human life, and that there is no morally relevant difference between the various developmental stages of a human life, human embryos must be treated with the same respect as any other human being.

There is another possible use for such embryos. Instead of being destroyed or used in research, they may be donated or sold to another couple whose infertility problems are even greater. Suppose, for example, that neither husband nor wife can contribute healthy gametes for a desperately desired child. Yet the wife is capable of becoming pregnant and bearing a child. In what might be labeled "prenatal adoption," it would be possible for an embryo resulting from IVF involving gametes of another couple to be placed in the wife's uterus. She could then experience the pregnancy and give birth to an "adopted" child. Although this use of frozen embryos may seem to many less repugnant than destroying them or using them in research, the technology that makes it possible also allows for other, more controversial combinations of genetic, biological, and social parenthood.

With ordinary human reproduction, AIH, and the standard case of IVF and EP, there is no difference between genetic and social parenthood. Those whose gametes combine to form a child and those who rear it are one and the same. AID, however, introduces a distinction between the genetic father (the sperm donor) and the social or legal father (the husband of the impregnated woman). It also permits a similar distinction between the genetic and gestational mother (a so-called surrogate mother) and the social mother, when the surrogate agrees (often through a contract and for a fee) to become pregnant through AID with the husband's sperm, to go through pregnancy, and then to give the infant to the husband and wife soon after it is born. The possibilities multiply in the context of IVF. Consider, for example, a child conceived in vitro from the sperm of A and the egg of B (the genetic parents), placed in the uterus of C (the gestational parent), and immediately after birth taken home and raised as the child of D and E (the social parents).

Moreover, none of these parties need be related to each other as legal husband and wife (D and E might even be a homosexual or lesbian couple). An even more bizarre possibility has recently been suggested (though not endorsed) by an Australian professor of obstetrics and gynecology: "[A]n embryo could be transferred to the peritoneal cavity of a male to female transexual and might in the presence of adequate hormonal stimulation grow adequately within the peritoneal cavity as an abdominal pregnancy resulting eventually in the birth of a normal living child by abdominal delivery" (1: p. 19). This would be tantamount to a male pregnancy.

What Should Be Done?

Responses to these new ways of creating human life have ranged from alarmist calls for total prohibition at one extreme to considerably more permissive attitudes at the other. In between are a number of positions that emphasize varying degrees of legal regulation. These usually include specifying the legal mother and father of children whose social parents are not identical with their genetic or gestational "parents," determining the extent to which the procedures may be put to commercial purposes, and setting the parameters for embryo research. A primary concern of those urging regulation is the welfare of the children. "At all levels," as George Annas puts it, "the primary focus should be on protecting the interests of the children, even if their protection sometimes comes at the expense of some infertile couples. This general policy will also protect the integrity of artificial reproduction itself" (2: p. 52).

Underlying current debates over which type of response is most adequate are a number of complex ethical issues. Although we cannot do justice to them here, we want to identify and briefly discuss three of them: 1) conflicting conceptions of parenthood and the family; 2) conflicting obligations of health professionals to patients, prospective children, and society, coupled with a concern for their own personal and professional integrity; and 3) conflicting conceptions of the nature and value of human embryos.

Parenthood and the Family

Apart from AIH and the standard case of IVF and EP, the new technologies for overcoming infertility seem to breed confusion by emphasizing the possibility of three types of parenthood—genetic, gestational, and social—where before (with the exception of standard cases of adoption) there was only one. Should we welcome these new possibilities or deplore and resist them? What are their implications for our idea of the family, and how will they affect children?

Advocates of the embattled traditional family oppose separating social from genetic and gestational parenthood, except for carefully regulated conventional adoption. The Catholic Church, for example, has taken a stand against surrogate parenting that closely follows its position against contraception. Sexuality, procreation, and parenthood, the Church maintains, are all part of the same fabric and must, with the exception of conventional adoption, be closely connected. Others, who may not agree with Catholic prohibitions of contraception, share the Church's worries about the future of the traditional family. Weakened by a high divorce rate, spiraling increases in teenage pregnancy, and a more permissive attitude toward unwed motherhood, the traditional family makes up a smaller proportion of households than it did in the past. And the new reproductive technology may further contribute to its decline.

A single woman who has no wish to be married, but who would like to bear and rear children, may, for example, turn to AID to become pregnant. Similarly, a lesbian couple may approach an *in vitro* fertilization clinic with an unusual request: they want to have an egg taken from one of them; have it fertilized with sperm from an anonymous donor; and then placed in the womb of the other, who would bear the child. In this way they would each have a biological connection with the child, one genetic and the other gestational. Variations on this theme involving a single man or a homosexual couple are also possible. Thus a consenting woman could serve as both genetic and gestational mother after being impregnated via AID with sperm from either the single man or one of the homosexual couple. Then, after the birth of the child, either the man or the homosexual couple would assume full social parenthood.

Defenders of the traditional family are usually opposed to these and similar possibilities. Not only do they regard these new types of "family" as harmful to society as a whole (largely because they believe that such "families" undermine the strength of the traditional family, society's bedrock), but they also think that such "families" will be harmful to children born into them. These new types of families, so the argument goes, cannot provide a minimally decent environment for a child. Therefore, aiding and abetting—or even tolerating—the use of various techniques for overcoming infertility to allow single women or men or lesbian or homosexual couples to start families is to place the interests of selfish, perhaps immoral, adults above those of the innocent children who would, as a result, be harmed.

Those who wish to make unorthodox use of the new reproductive techniques may respond by pointing out that changing attitudes toward divorce and unwed motherhood, as well as various social and economic changes, have already resulted in an increasing number of children being born or raised outside of traditional, two-parent families. If so many other single persons or unmarried couples are permitted to have and raise children, they may ask, why shouldn't they be allowed to use the new technology to do the same? The desire to become a parent, after all, has deep biological and cultural roots. Moreover, there is a presumption in Anglo-American legal systems against interfering with a person's reproductive desires or capacity unless it is necessary to prevent demonstrable harm. As Somerville has recently suggested about the use of AID by lesbian couples, "It makes a difference whether artificial insemination is refused to a person simply because of that person's sexual orientation or because of the potential harm of that sexual orientation to the child who will be born. The latter is probably justifiable, the former may not be" (3: p. 133). Thus unless it can be shown that the use of this new technology by single women and gay couples is likely to cause excessive harm to children or to society, it may be a form of prejudice or discrimination to prohibit them from using it.

Will a child conceived through AID, with or without IVF and EP, and then raised by a single mother be adversely affected? Will a male born to a lesbian couple be more likely to become homosexual or be poorly raised than a child born to a heterosexual couple? Will the fabric of society be weakened if homosexual couples are allowed to "have" children with the cooperation of a consenting gestational mother and AID? The resolution of the conflict between defenders of the traditional family and those wanting to employ the new reproductive technologies in unorthodox ways turns on the answers to questions such as these.

Although there is more to be learned about these matters, reviews of the relevant social science research suggest that arguments against AID for single women based on harm to the children are not supported by the available data (4, 5). If this is correct, there may be no basis for a blanket prohibition of AID for single women. Strong and Schinfeld have accordingly proposed that decisions about AID for single women be made case by case (4). They set out and illustrate guidelines to help physicians evaluate requests from single women which reflect an informed concern for the welfare of the prospective child as well as a desire to take the requests seriously.

Strong and Schinfeld advise physicians to determine the patient's physical and financial capacities for rearing a child, and to undertake counseling with regard to such matters as the importance of child-adult interaction, the advisability of an immediate or extended family for support, and so on. To illustrate their recommendation, they sketch a case of a 40-year-old executive who had never been married who requested AID. She had a regular male sexual partner and impregnation by him was an alternative, but she did not want to marry or to share the raising of a child with him. She was in good health, financially quite well off, and had the support of her family and a supporting letter from a psychiatrist. After further investigation and counseling, the authors concluded that it was reasonable for a physician to fulfill her request.

Other types of request may, however, be more difficult to evaluate. For example, although the available evidence does not suggest significant harm to children raised by a lesbian parent, the number of relevant studies is limited and there are even fewer data available on children raised by lesbian or homosexual couples. Requests for the new reproductive technologies by such parties may, therefore, be more problematic than those of single, heterosexual women who want to become parents but who have no desire to marry or to share the raising of a child with a man. Still, it is not clear that such requests can be categorically rejected.

In short, the debate is fraught with moral complexity and empirical uncertainty. Concerns about the effect of new forms of human reproduction on the family and on society cannot be lightly dismissed. At the same time, it is difficult to support an absolute prohibition of unorthodox uses of AID, IVF, and EP as long as there are no restrictions on single parenting in general and the anticipated ill effects are not yet substantiated. Our presumption of privacy and liberty with regard to reproduction cannot be overridden without strong evidence of the likelihood of harm. In the meantime we might consider extending Strong and Schinfeld's thoughtful guidelines for case-by-case evaluation of requests for AID by single women to cover all unorthodox requests for the new technology, at least until new evidence or arguments are produced to justify some other course.

Obligation and Integrity

To say that it may in certain cases be permissible to employ AID, IVF, and EP to enable single women or lesbian couples to become parents is not, however, to say that it is obligatory. The same is true of less controversial uses of the new technology, including, for example, variations of IVF and EP involving participants other than a husband and wife. Thus physicians who are troubled or unsure about the ethical complexities or social implications of the new reproductive technologies are not obligated to use them (6). Appeals to one's personal or professional integrity are sufficient to justify a refusal to honor or even to consider ethically controversial requests for AID, IVF, and EP.

A reluctant physician can readily acknowledge that many unmarried women have babies (some are even doing so with the cooperation of a consenting male friend and "do-it-yourself" AID [3]), and that some lesbians and homosexuals retain custody of their children after divorce or the deaths of their spouses. Such a physician may even acknowledge that many of these turn out to be good parents and that their children appear to be doing well. At the same time he or she may consistently refuse to be a party to unorthodox uses of the new reproductive technology. That these things happen and that some of them turn out well is one thing; that a particular physician has to be a party to them is quite another. As a matter of conscience, personal values, or his or her conception of the nature and function of medicine, a physician may justifiably refuse to honor ethically controversial requests for the new reproductive technology.

It is important, however, that such justifiable appeals to conscience be carefully distinguished from unsupportable claims about the invariable ill effects of such practices or the unqualified condemnation of all those who engage in them. As suggested above, we cannot show that all unorthodox uses of the new technology will have harmful effects; nor is it true that all who participate in such uses, be they patients or physicians, are thoughtless or unconcerned about ethical or social implications. There is room for reasonable disagreement on these matters as evidenced, perhaps, by a survey, published in 1979, in which 9.5 percent of those physicians responding indicated that they had used AID on single women (7). But a physician confronted with a request for one or another form of the new reproductive technology who is understandably troubled by what appear to be conflicting obligations to patients, prospective children, and society may, on this basis alone, justifiably refuse to comply with it. The grounds for what has come to be called "conscientious refusal" are weaker than those needed to interfere with or condemn others who are doing what one cannot, in good conscience, do oneself.

Status of Human Embryos

As mentioned above, a number of frozen embryos may be left over after a couple has made standard use of IVF and EP and plans to have no more children. What should be done with the surplus embryos? Putting aside for the moment the question of whether they may be donated or sold to another infertile couple or to a single woman, may they be either washed down the drain or used in research? Those who believe that life begins at conception and that all human life is equally sacred would emphatically answer "No." Throwing the embryos away would be tantamount to murder, and using them as subjects of experiments would be to do so without their informed consent. Others, however, take a different view. Although they may concede that a human embryo is a living human being, they will deny that is is sufficiently developed in terms of central nervous system activity, sentience, self-awareness, self-determination, or some other (set of) characteristic(s) to come under the protection of moral or legal prohibitions against murder or against being subjects in important, well-designed (and painless) research. At the center of this controversy are questions about the moral and metaphysical status of human embryos.

This is a matter that lies at the heart of many of the ethical issues considered in this book. Not only embryos, but also fetuses at various stages of development, and even newborn infants differ in important respects from somewhat older children or adults. If asked why the latter have a *right* to life—why, that is, they *themselves* would *be wronged* by being killed or deprived of life-sustaining treatment—we would probably base our response, in part, on their capacity for self-awareness and their sense of the future. As Kuhse and Singer have put it: "A self-aware being with a sense of the future can have hopes and desires about what might or might not happen to it in the future. To kill it is to prevent the fulfillment of these hopes and desires" (8: p. 120). But a being that cannot understand that it exists as a separate being, that has no plans, projects, or intentions for the future, cannot, they maintain, be similarly wronged. If this is correct, it is not so clear that simply being a member of our species or having the potential to develop a capacity for self-awareness and a sense of the future, or both, are sufficient to endow a human embryo, fetus, or severely premature or seriously ill newborn with a *right* to life. But does it also follow that, say, a human embryo has no independent value or standing at all? If a being does not (yet) have a capacity for self-awareness and a sense of the future, may we do with it whatever we will as long as the results promise to be of benefit?

The Warnock Committee on Human Fertilization and Embryology in Great Britain has addressed this question in the context of embryo research. The question was whether and, if so, to what extent, well-designed scientific research could be conducted on human embryos created by IVF. How, that is, should the value of a human embryo be weighed against the significant advantages to society and future parents and children of using it as a research subject? Those who regarded the embryo as having the same status as, say, ordinary children or adults were opposed to any such research, for an embryo is in no position to give its informed consent to it. Those who regarded not only embryos, but also fetuses, as having a quite different status from children or adults, thought the research should be regulated only by scientific considerations.

The Warnock Committee appears to have taken a moderate or middle-of-the-road position on this issue. Focusing on the importance of the formation of the primitive streak in the development of the human individual, a majority of the Committee recommended that "no live human embryo derived from *in vitro* fertilization, whether frozen or unfrozen, may be kept alive, if not transferred to a woman, beyond 14 days after fertilization, nor may it be used as a research subject beyond 14 days after fertilization. This 14-day period does not include any time during which the embryo may have been frozen" (9: p. 66). A minority of three of the Committee's 16 members dissented from this recommendation. Emphasizing the embryo's *potential* for developing into a human person, the minority argued that it is wrong to create an entity with the potential for developing into a human person and then destroying it. Their recommendation was that "nothing should be done that would reduce the chance of successful implantation of the embryo" and that "experimentation on the human embryo is not permitted" (9: p. 90f).

Inasmuch as the underlying philosophical issue here arises both during pregnancy, with regard to questions of abortion and fetal surgery, and shortly after birth, with regard to questions of how aggressively to treat severely premature or seriously ill newborns, we will examine these aspects in subsequent sections and defer normative recommendation until the section on public policy.

Genetic Assessment

Genetic assessment cuts across the three developmental periods that provide the organizational focus of this overview and the book as a whole. Certain forms of genetic screening, such as, for example, large-scale efforts to identify those at risk for bearing children with Tay-Sachs disease or sickle cell anemia, occur before implantation. Prenatal diagnosis, perhaps the most traumatic and momentous form of genetic assessment, is currently restricted to a certain segment of the intrauterine period. And other forms of genetic screening, such as testing newborns for phenylketonuria (PKU), occur during the postnatal period. Some forms of genetic assessment involve two or more of these periods. For example, counseling that includes determining the likelihood of a couple's having a second baby with a certain genetic anomaly takes place after the birth of the affected child and while the couple is contemplating the conception of another. In what follows we will emphasize the preimplantation period. Issues that arise primarily in the intrauterine period will be discussed in the next section. Chapter 3, John Fletcher's wide-ranging and comprehensive discussion of genetic assessment, covers all three periods.

A couple whose child is born with a genetic disease or anomaly may well want to know their chances of having a second child with the same problem. If they regard the risks as too high, they may consider not having more children, completing their family through adoption, or, depending on the source of the defective gene, AID or some variation of IVF and EP. It is the role of the genetic counselor to help the parents think these matters through. He or she should know enough about medical genetics to provide them with accurate, intelligible information about the nature and likelihood of the relevant genetic disease or anomaly. At the same time the genetic counselor should be skilled in helping parents sort through the relevant factors and to arrive at an informed decision that reflects their considered judgments about values, desires, psychological and financial resources, and so on. This aspect of genetic counseling requires careful judgment. One has to avoid the twin pitfalls of imposing one's own values and preferences, on the one hand, and being overly distant and detached, on the other. Whether, and if so to what extent, genetic counselors can or should walk this delicate line is still a matter of debate.

Among the ethical dilemmas confronting genetic counselors, those involving confidentiality are especially difficult and troubling. What should be done when a client refuses to allow genetic information to be shared with relatives who are also likely to be at risk? The venerable, well-grounded duty of confidentiality requires respecting the client's wishes, yet the equally plausible duty of beneficence requires that the information be disclosed. A related problem arises when the results of a genetic analysis strongly suggest that the ostensible father of a child with a genetic illness is not the biological father, and the required counseling cannot take place without this being disclosed. Does the counselor provide the relevant information at the cost of risking the marriage or relationship? Or does the counselor try to preserve the relationship by euphemistically reporting the findings?

Some couples may be directed to or may seek genetic counseling before having their first child. If, for example, past occurrence of genetic anomalies in one or both blood lines suggests a greater than average risk for an affected child, the couple may want additional information, guidance, and reassurance before deciding to have a child of their own. More controversial, from an ethical point of view, are screening programs that attempt to identify unsuspecting carriers of certain congenital illnesses, in some cases even before the couple are married.

Various types of screening programs have been conducted to identify carriers of certain diseases in high-risk populations; for example, Tay-Sachs disease among Ashkenazic Jews, sickle cell disease in blacks, and thalessemia among members of certain communities of Mediterranean extraction. At their inception a number of these programs were, as Fletcher points out in Chapter 3, premature, harmful, and coercive. They proceeded without adequate understanding of the nature of the relevant disease, stigmatized and caused gratuitous worry among and discrimination against those identified as carriers, and ignored considerations of informed consent. Although guidelines have since been formulated to exclude the most egregious abuses, genetic screening remains ethically problematic. Should screening for certain illnesses be voluntary or mandatory? What pressures will be brought to bear on those who have been identified to be at high risk and yet still intend to bear children? Would third-party payers be justified in withholding benefits in such cases? As funding for medical care becomes both more restricted and shared (through government programs, health insurance, health maintenance organizations, and so on) and as we develop the medical capacities to identify heterozygotes for a larger number of congenital conditions, such questions will become unavoidable. These problems are magnified if screening is proposed as a condition of employment. We can understand how attempts to reduce the increasing cost of medical insurance may tempt employers to identify and reject applicants whose employment would place them at additional risk for bearing congenitally ill children, but is this justifiable?

These and related questions about the legitimate uses of ever more powerful and comprehensive techniques of genetic assessment require thoughtful and informed analysis and discussion. They will not go away. Like AID, IVF, and EP, new forms of genetic assessment can be employed in ways other than those envisaged by the scientists and physicians who developed them. Parents, prospective parents, health professionals, and policymakers must now try to distinguish the more from less justifiable uses of these new techniques.

Intrauterine Period

Some issues that arise prior to implantation assume new forms during the intrauterine period. Genetic assessment, undertaken either through amniocentesis or perhaps chorionic biopsy, now involves an actual, and not simply a contemplated, pregnancy. Questions about contraception become questions about abortion, and debates about the moral standing of embryos that arise in discussions of IVF metamorphize into more heated controversies about the moral standing of the fetus. Equally troubling, from an ethical point of view, are conflicts between the interests of a fetus that is not going to be aborted and the personal interests or autonomy of the mother. These conflicts have recently been sharpened by new information about the relationships between certain kinds of maternal behavior (for example, heavy smoking, drinking, or drug use) and fetal well-being and by interventions, such as fetal therapy, fetal surgery, and cesarean delivery, that are undertaken to optimize the health of the fetus at some additional risk or discomfort to the mother. What responsibilities or duties does a pregnant woman have to her developing fetus? How are we to resolve conflicts between the mother's autonomy and bodily integrity, on the one hand, and what is believed to be in the fetus's best interests, on the other? This set of problems becomes more difficult still, we might note, when the gestational mother (the pregnant woman) is not expected to be the social mother and may or may not be the genetic mother. In cases like this, made possible by the new reproductive technology, who should be authorized to make decisions about chorionic biopsy, amniocentesis, abortion, drinking, smoking, drug use, prenatal care, eating habits, fetal therapy, and whether to have a cesarean or a vaginal delivery? Should it be the gestational (or surrogate) mother or the prospective social parents?

Prenatal Diagnosis

The capacity to identify an increasing number of genetic diseases in utero remains controversial largely because of the inability to treat most of them. The usual response to prenatally detected genetic disease is to abort the affected fetus. Yet abortions for genetic indications are, in some ways, more problematic than abortions for pregnancies that are wholly unwanted.

First, given the present state of the art, a diagnosis of one or another genetic disease cannot be confirmed through amniocentesis until well into the second trimester of pregnancy. Abortions, in such cases, are usually performed between week 18 and week 21 of gestation. A fetus at this stage is significantly more highly developed than an embryo or a fetus during the first trimester of pregnancy. Its central nervous system and various organs and organ systems are drawing very near to the stages of development of some premature infants who are now benefiting from advances in neonatal care. Moreover, since the pregnancy is

generally intended and a child wanted, an abortion at this stage is psychologically quite hard on the parents. It is also more difficult technically
than an earlier abortion. Each of the three more or less standard methods of late abortion is problematic. Intra-amniotic injection of concen-
trated saline solution guarantees the death of the fetus but provides
certain risks to the mother. Inducing labor by use of prostaglandins
provides a lower risk to the mother's health but does not guarantee that
the fetus will die, and some fetuses that survive labor can be liveborn.
Dilation and evacuation (D&E), while safe for the mother and ensuring
death of the fetus, requires greater skill on the part of the physician, and
because it requires explicit dismemberment of the fetus, it is an understandably repugnant procedure for many medical professionals (10).

The development of chorionic villus sampling, as an alternative to
amniocentesis, would mitigate some of these problems by providing for
the detection of the same genetic illnesses at a much earlier stage of
pregnancy. At this time, however, the procedure is experimental, and
its safety and accuracy as compared to amniocentesis are still being
studied (11). Even if chorionic villus sampling proves to be as safe and
accurate as amniocentesis and thus eliminates some of the problems
posed by late abortion, many who are strongly opposed to abortion for
genetic indications will not be satisfied by earlier detection and hence
earlier abortion. Their objection to abortions of this kind is based on
principles that are independent of the stages of fetal development.

Although a recent public opinion poll indicates that abortions intended to prevent the birth of a genetically deformed or handicapped
child are acceptable to 64 percent of the American public (12), Kristen
Luker has pointed out that abortions for "fetal indications" are among
those least tolerable, ideologically, for those who are actively opposed to
legalized abortion:

[A]bortions for fetal deformity cut to the deepest level of pro-life feeling about
"selective abortion." Because the logic of abortion in this case depends upon a
judgment that the embryo is "damaged" in one respect or another, it suggests to
pro-life people an acceptance of the idea that humans can be ranked along some
scale of perfection and that people who fall below a certain arbitrary standard
can be excluded. . . . Already, for example, the movement is vigorously opposing amniocentesis. . . . The present surgeon-general of the United States,
[C.] Everett Koop, an active pro-life supporter, has called amniocentesis exams
"search and destroy missions," and the movement itself has labeled amniocentesis "selective genocide against the disabled" (13: p. 236).

A similar outlook can be found among some advocates for the disabled
who, though generally supporting *Roe v. Wade*, are opposed to abortion

for "fetal indications," because, they maintain, it suggests that the disabled are less valuable than other people.

In addressing this line of argument, there is no avoiding the question of the moral status of the fetus. If the fetus has the same moral standing as a typical adult human, the pro-life argument against abortion for fetal indications will in most cases be quite difficult to refute. For if one cannot justifiably take steps to end the life of an adult with Down syndrome or cystic fibrosis, neither should one be able to do so with a similarly affected fetus. Abortion for "fetal indications" will, at most, only be justified for a small number of severe anomalies, such as anencephaly. Those who oppose this restrictive position must, therefore, provide an alternative account of the moral status of the fetus, one that is both plausible and compatible with their more permissive views of abortion. This, however, is more difficult than many of them suppose.

Moral Status of the Fetus

There are three main positions on the moral status of the fetus. The first, what we will call the "extreme conservative position," focuses on human life *as such* and therefore emphasizes the similarities, as living human beings, between postnatal human beings, who clearly fall under the protection of laws against murder, and prenatal human beings. For the extreme conservative, human life begins at conception and all living human beings are (or should be) equally protected by laws against killing. The second position, what we will call the "extreme liberal position," emphasizes the secular reasons we are inclined to give when asked to explain why killing humans, from an ethical point of view, is much worse than, say, killing animals. Most humans, as opposed to most (if not all) animals, have interests and desires for the future and various plans and projects that cannot be fulfilled unless they remain alive. Therefore, the loss *to them* if they are killed is much greater than that to (most?) animals. Extrapolating from this, the extreme liberal then maintains that the right to life, and thus the right to be protected by laws against killing, does not become applicable until a being develops the capacities for self-awareness and a sense of the future; and this occurs *at the very earliest* shortly after birth. The third position, what we will call the "moderate position," falls in between the two extremes. For the moderate the fetus acquires independent moral standing some time after conception, the point favored by the extreme conservative, but before developing the comparatively sophisticated mental capacities required for independent moral standing by the extreme liberal. Although each of these positions has something to recommend it, none is free of serious difficulty.

The main trouble with the extreme conservative position is that it seems to prove too much. Taken seriously, it would, as Joel Feinberg has observed, require us to do as much to preserve the life of a newly fertilized ovum as for anyone else whose life is in danger (14: pp. 288–291). Over 40 percent of fertilized ova fail to survive until implantation, and the spontaneous abortion rate after implantation ranges from 10 to 20 percent. If we were to regard the life of an embryo or zygote as valuable as that of any postnatal human being, we would have to commit as much money and research effort to preventing this loss of human life as we commit to preventing the deaths of persons after they are born. Are those who espouse the extreme conservative position actually prepared to do this? Consider, too, that even if we were able to discover some sort of wonder drug that would save all of these human lives, most of which would be seriously handicapped, the incidence of congenital disease in the population would grow from approximately 2 percent suffering from relatively major congenital defects to over 20 percent who would suffer from a number of serious and incapacitating defects. Finally, defenders of the extreme conservative position are hard pressed to provide a plausible, *secular* explanation as to why all human life *as such* is equally valuable. The most likely secular argument would combine an emphasis on the consequences of our actions with a concern about embarking on a slippery slope: for example, "Once we allow the taking of any innocent human life, regardless of level of development, respect for the value of all human life will be eroded and no one will be safe." But the empirical evidence necessary to substantiate this worry has not been forthcoming. Advocates of the extreme conservative position are more likely to base their outlooks on explicitly or implicitly held theological outlooks or world views that place special value on human life as God's creation. These outlooks or world views are often quite attractive and worthy of our respect. But inasmuch as other equally plausible and respect-worthy theological and secular outlooks and world views differ with them on this matter, such defenses of the extreme conservative position cannot be regarded as morally binding on everyone in a nontheocratic, pluralistic society (14).

The main weakness of the extreme conservative position—its inability to provide a plausible secular explanation as to why the taking of all human life is equally wrong—becomes the main strength of the extreme liberal position. By focusing on the fundamental importance for each of us of our intentions, plans, and projects for the future, the extreme liberal can explain why, as individuals, we generally fear death and regard killing as the ultimate evil; death (or at least a premature death) deprives us of everything that we want. And since even an irascible hermit can be supposed to have intentions, plans, and projects, killing him would be wrong even if no one would miss him or even learn of his death. Nevertheless, the extreme liberal position suffers from a major embarrassment. Like the extreme conservative position it, too, seems to prove too much, though in the opposite direction. For it appears to allow not only early abortion, but also late-term abortion and even infanticide and the killing of the very severely retarded and senile. This is because neither late-term fetuses nor infants nor at least some of the severely retarded and senile will have the cognitive capacities to frame intentions and make plans and projects for the future. Like most nonhuman animals their lives will be governed by instinct and the perception of the immediate present. Proponents of the extreme liberal position are aware of this difficulty and have tried to respond to it, but the cogency of their efforts remains in dispute (15–17).

Moderates seize upon the counterintuitive consequences of both extreme positions. According to moderates, the conservative grants a fetus the right to life too early and the liberal too late; the conservative's position on abortion is therefore too restrictive and the liberal's too permissive. The moral status of the fetus becomes weighty enough to prohibit killing and abortion, the moderate maintains, somewhere in between the two extremes. But exactly where? And for what reasons? This is where the moderate view founders. Each of the most plausible candidates—for example, central nervous system activity, quickening, sentience, viability, and birth—is criticized, with good reason, as morally arbitrary by liberals and conservatives alike (16–18). It is hard to understand, the critics argue, why any of these differences is significant enough, from an ethical point of view, to make a difference between life and death. Sophisticated moderates are aware of these difficulties and try to respond to them, but none has been notably successful (19).

Thus the moral status of the fetus remains problematic. The debate is likely to continue, but prospects for a widely accepted, well-grounded philosophical resolution, at least in the near future, are dim. Matters become even more complicated when one takes into account the larger social and economic context in which the philosophical debates take place. We cannot, for example, overlook the importance for the political activists on both sides of the question of competing conceptions of the nature and role of motherhood in contemporary society (13). Whether we can in the meantime work out a reasonably plausible and stable political accommodation among the contending parties will be taken up later in this chapter.

Conflicts Between Mother and Wanted Fetus

Although most pregnant woman are prepared to go to great lengths to maximize the well-being of their wanted fetuses, new information about the connection between various forms of maternal behavior and fetal development, as well as about the development of riskier and more invasive types of medical intervention, raises difficult questions about the nature and limits of maternal responsibility. Must a woman undergo any additional degree of pain, risk, discomfort, or inconvenience to assure optimal health for her soon-to-be-born child? Or are there limits as to what she can reasonably be required to do? And what is the relationship between ethical and legal responsibility? Can, for example, the coercive power of the state be brought to bear on those women who are not prepared to make certain kinds of sacrifices for the sake of their developing fetuses? These questions, though not entirely new, assume new urgency with recent advances in medical knowledge and technology.

Maintaining a healthy diet, seeking and complying with adequate prenatal care, and refraining from smoking, excessive drinking, and the use of various recreational drugs are all likely to contribute to the health of a developing fetus at comparably little risk, discomfort, or inconvenience to the mother. Women with certain sorts of illnesses may also have to take special precautions during pregnancy. For example, those with phenylketonuria will have to observe special (and unpleasant) dietary restrictions, while those with diabetes will have to make sure that they keep their disease under control (20). The likelihood and degree of harm to the infant vary considerably. Although the possibility of a PKU mother who fails to follow the prescribed dietary restrictions giving birth to a mentally retarded child are practically 100 percent, the likelihood and severity of harm to the infant from, say, maternal smoking or drinking, are less certain. Still, most of us regard reducing the risk of various harms to the fetus that may last a lifetime as much more important than a woman's refraining from certain pleasurable behaviors or adopting certain unpleasant or inconvenient behaviors for the duration of her pregnancy. But what can we do about those who appear to balance the competing values differently?

First we must try to understand exactly why the mother is acting as she is. Does she fully understand the magnitude and degree of risk? Are there special social, cultural, psychological, or financial considerations that are governing her behavior? One may then want to undertake various forms of education, rational persuasion, and, if these are not fully effective, certain forms of coaxing, cajoling, and even scolding and chastizing, depending upon the mother's background and character. Much as one may be tempted to do so, however, resort to the courts or seeking additional legal sanctions are, in this instance, ethically questionable and likely to be of limited value. As Fleischman and Macklin point out in Chapter 5, the risks to the fetus are usually too uncertain to justify the all too certain harm of legal interference with an autonomous adult. Moreover, laws restricting maternal behavior during the entire course of pregnancy will be almost impossible to enforce without either incarcerating offenders for the duration of pregnancy or adopting invasions of privacy characteristic of a police state.

Fetal therapy, as opposed to altering maternal behavior, is concerned with relatively brief stages of pregnancy. But the contemplated interventions are much more invasive. Perhaps the most well-established and least controversial form of fetal therapy is intrauterine blood transfusion to correct a potentially lethal Rh incompatibility between mother and fetus. More recently, intrauterine exchange transfusions through the umbilical vein have been successfully performed (21). Here the risk to the mother is slight and the benefit to the fetus very great. The main difficulty from an ethical point of view has to do with court orders compelling such treatment when the mother is a Jehovah's Witness and therefore strongly opposed to the transfusion of blood. Other forms of therapy have been proposed for certain defects detected *in utero* by prenatal diagnosis. They include surgical correction for such conditions as hydronephrosis, diaphragmatic hernia, and hydrocephalus. At the moment, however, these proposed interventions are still quite experimental and characterized by a great deal of uncertainty. If and when they become perfected they are likely to raise difficult conflicts. Fetal surgery is also a surgical intervention for the mother and requires her consent as an involved party, not simply as a proxy for the fetus. What, then, should we do if a particular surgical intervention on and for the fetus, but through the mother, will provide nearly certain and significant benefit to the fetus, but involve a significant degree of risk, pain, and suffering to the mother? Whose interests are paramount in a case like this and why?

Some of the questions raised by the prospect of nonexperimental fetal surgery are already with us in the context of childbirth. The issue is whether and, if so, under what circumstances, a woman can be forced to undergo a cesarean rather than a vaginal delivery. Courts in at least two states have already ordered women who were refusing surgical interventions during labor to undergo them. Can this be justified? The risk of death to a mother during cesarean delivery is four times that of vaginal delivery. If a woman can rightfully be coerced into taking this additional risk, why stop with childbirth? Why not also require mothers (and fathers) to undertake the risks of surgery or general anesthesia in order to donate bone marrow or a kidney to a dying child (22)? In fact the courts do not order such interventions, and with good reason, even though we admire and commend parents who make such sacrifices for their children.

The right to bodily integrity and the requirement of informed consent as a necessary condition for medical interventions are important elements of our way of life that should not be lightly disregarded. Once we begin going to court to order one person to undergo surgery for the benefit of another, where will we stop? Although we can understand the consternation of physicians whose concern for the welfare of fetuses and infants is frustrated by what they regard as unreasonable refusals of cesarean delivery, we suggest that they reflect on the wider implications of going to court. The overwhelming majority of women, as noted above, are inclined to make significant sacrifices for their children, especially when they are reliably and respectfully informed of the probable consequences of their behavior. Although respecting maternal autonomy may, in rare cases, result in avoidable deaths or defects for fetuses, this may, on balance, be the less harmful alternative when we consider the more far-reaching consequences of overriding the right to bodily integrity and the requirement of informed consent (22).

Conflicts Among Parents

Many of the foregoing issues become even more difficult if the pregnancy is a product of the new reproductive technology and the gestational mother is a surrogate for another person or couple planning to become the social parent(s). Consider, for example, a situation where the pregnant woman, a surrogate mother, is strongly urged, for the sake of the fetus and its future welfare, to undergo a cesarean delivery, but she is reluctant to run the additional risks of surgery. Whose voice should be stronger here, hers or that of the prospective social parents? Similar conflicts are possible with regard to the other issues we have identified in this section. If, for example, the gestational mother is not identical with the social mother, who is to have the last word as to whether the former should be allowed to smoke, drink, or take certain recreational drugs during her pregnancy? And whatever agreements are struck about these and related matters, how are they to be enforced?

Parental conflict, it is important to note, is not restricted to situations involving surrogate pregnancy. Differences between mother and father can also arise during the course of a conventional pregnancy. Suppose a decision has to be made as to whether to undertake a treatment that would have some desirable benefit for the fetus but would significantly increase the mother's risk of death or otherwise impair her health. Suppose, too, that the mother's selfless concern for the welfare of the fetus is so strong that she is more than willing to run the additional risk to herself. Her husband, however, is of a different opinion. He is understandably concerned about their two young children and the difficulties that could arise if they became motherless. He is also more interested for his own sake in the welfare of his wife than of the prospective child. If husband and wife cannot come to some kind of agreement in such a case, whose wishes should weigh most heavily with the physicians and why?

There may be many variations on this theme. Consider a similar situation in which the benefits to the fetus of a particular intervention would be great and the risks to the mother very small; yet in this instance the mother is reluctant to place herself at additional risk. If the father was strongly in favor of the procedure and urged the physician to undertake it for the sake of the fetus, how much weight should be given to his views?

Although the mother is the one who is pregnant, the role of the father with regard to ethical issues during pregnancy is likely to demand increased attention. This owes, in part, to the increased emphasis that the women's movement has rightfully placed on the procreative and parental responsibilities of males. As we come to recognize the father's greater responsibility both for conception and for the care of the infant after it is born, we cannot deny him a significant role in decision making during the course of pregnancy. But the biological differences between men and women with regard to pregnancy—and its risks, discomforts, and inconveniences—will not allow the roles to be entirely equal or provide an easy way of reconciling certain types of disagreement.

Postnatal Period

Difficult questions about the status and treatment of seriously ill newborns remain unanswered despite attempts in the United States to settle the matter through federal regulation. Although the recently effected "Baby Doe regulations" (23) will undoubtedly affect subsequent debate, they will not eliminate it (24, 25). As with the Supreme Court's *Roe v. Wade* decision on abortion (1973), ethical controversies remain despite efforts to settle them at the levels of constitutional law or federal policy. Underlying the ethical debate are three interrelated questions (26). First, should a seriously ill newborn (or, for that matter, any infant) be regarded as having the same moral and legal status as a normal adult human? This is a postnatal version of our earlier questions about the status of the embryo and the fetus. Second, to what extent, if any, and for what reasons, if any, are judgments about the quality of an infant's life relevant to decisions about how aggressively to sustain that life? Some argue that judgments of this kind are impossible, while others maintain, with equal conviction, that they are unavoidable. And third, what role should the burdens of raising and providing for a seriously handicapped child be allowed to play in the decision making? While many believe that the possible effects of such a child on a family or on society are of no relevance for life-and-death decisions, others hold that they are of the greatest importance.

Moral Status of the Infant

"While one may empathize with the parents of a defective infant," John Robertson has written, "one cannot forget that the innocent life of an untreated child is also involved. Like any infant, the deformed child is a person with a right to life—a right that is the basis of our social order and legal system" (27: p. 216). Those who share this view are likely to accord parents and physicians very little discretion in determining whether it is permissible to withhold or withdraw life-sustaining treatment from a seriously ill newborn. Only, perhaps, if the infant meets the following exceptions set out by the final rule governing the "withholding of medically indicated treatment from disabled infants with life-threatening conditions" implemented in April 1985 by the U.S. Department of Health and Human Services (23: p. 14878) would Robertson's position allow for the denial of treatment:

1. The infant is chronically and irreversibly comatose; or
2. The provision of such treatment would merely prolong dying, not be effective in ameliorating or correcting all of the infant's life-threatening conditions, or otherwise be futile in terms of the survival of the infant; or
3. The provision of such treatment would be virtually futile in terms of the survival of the infant and the treatment itself under such circumstances would be inhumane.

Yet many of us are likely to be ambivalent about such a restrictive position, even if we are initially attracted to the claim that "like any infant, the deformed child is a person with a right to life."

One indication of this ambivalence is, as Thomas H. Murray has observed, "the contrast between our outcry at the death of Baby Doe [the Bloomington, Indiana, newborn with Down syndrome who was allowed to die from unoperated esophageal atresia in 1982], and the approximately 90,000 amniocenteses done every year to detect genetic anomalies like trisomy 21—Down syndrome—in pregnant women aged 35 and older" (28: p. 9). The tests alone, Murray adds, cost over $50 million and result in 500 to 800 abortions of Down syndrome fetuses per year. Is the difference between fetus and newborn strong enough to merit this contrast? Extreme conservatives maintain that it is not, and consequently argue for prohibitions on aborting fetuses, as well as for mandatory treatment of infants with, for example, Down syndrome and most other anomalies at birth. Some extreme liberals turn this position inside out. Building upon a very permissive position on abortion, they suggest that the metaphysical status of a newborn with, say, Down syndrome differs little from that of a similarly affected fetus. If, therefore, it is permissible to abort such a fetus, it is also permissible to withhold life-sustaining treatment from a similarly affected newborn.

Underlying this outlook is the belief that a being cannot *itself* be wronged by death unless it has interests and desires about the future and various plans and projects that cannot be fulfilled unless it remains alive (29). Thus, the very same arguments that show that a fetus is not *itself* wronged by an abortion are sufficient, for some extreme liberals, to show that an infant is not *itself* wronged by being denied life-sustaining medical treatment. This is not, however, to endorse a wanton disregard for the lives of disabled infants. In their recent defense of an extreme liberal position, Kuhse and Singer (8) have identified a number of conditions that would significantly limit the number of infants from whom life-sustaining treatment could rightly be withheld or withdrawn, even if one maintains, as they do, that such infants do not have interests in, or a right to, continued life. A particular infant's potential for a happy and "worthwhile" life, the fact that most infants, even those born with disabilities, are very much wanted and loved by their parents, and the availability of adoptive or foster parents who would, if given the opportunity, cherish a disabled newborn and bring it up as their own, provide strong utilitarian grounds for protecting the lives of the vast majority of newborns, including many with certain disabilities (9). Life-sustaining treatment would be withheld, on Kuhse and Singer's extreme liberal position, only from those seriously ill newborns with little potential for a happy life, whose parents do not want to raise them, and for whom neither loving adoptive or foster parents nor optimal institutionalized care can be provided. Still, this position will be too permissive for extreme conservatives and the contingency of the restrictions is probably too weak to be acceptable to most moderates. Thus, the question of the moral status of the newborn, like that of the embryo and fetus, remains unsettled.

Quality of Life

A related controversy centers on the extent to which judgments about the "quality of life" may enter into decisions about withholding or withdrawing life-sustaining treatment from a handicapped infant. Those who, like Robertson, emphasize the equal value of each human life are extremely reluctant to compare the "quality" of the lives of otherwise normal persons with, say, those born with Down syndrome, spina bifida, low birthweight, and various other disabilities. In many cases, they maintain, such comparisons exaggerate the amount of pain and suffering associated with the impaired condition or else overlook the fact that with better social and parental support, the disability would become considerably less handicapping. Even at their strongest, Robertson maintains, quality-of-life arguments require, "a proxy's judgment that no reasonable person can prefer the pain, suffering, and loneliness of, for example, life in a crib at an IQ of 20 to a painless death" (27: p. 254). But such third-person judgments of quality are notoriously difficult to substantiate:

In what sense can the proxy validly conclude that a person with different wants, needs, and interests, if able to speak would agree that such a life were worse than death? . . . One who has never known the pleasures of mental operation, ambulation, and social interaction surely does not suffer from their loss as much as one who has. While one who has known these capacities may prefer death to a life without them, we have no assurance that the handicapped person, with no point of comparison would agree. Life, and life alone, whatever its limitations, might be of sufficient worth to him (27: p. 254).

Appeals to a low quality of life are most plausible, Robertson adds, "in the case of a grossly deformed, retarded, institutionalized child, or one with incessant unmanageable pain, where continued life is itself a torture." But because, he maintains, such cases are few and the dangers of opening up the door to quality-of-life judgments are many, we should categorically reject judgments about the quality of life as grounds for withholding or withdrawing life-sustaining treatment from seriously ill newborns.

This, however, is easier said than done. As newborn intensive care becomes ever more successful at sustaining life, the number of infants whose continued existence raises questions about the quality of their lives will grow larger and become more difficult to ignore for the sake of the greater overall good. Consider, for example, the three classes of exceptions, listed above, acknowledged by the U.S. government's final rule governing the treatment of disabled infants with life-threatening conditions. Despite protestations to the contrary, the Department of

Health and Human Services cannot provide a coherent defense of these exceptions without tacitly appealing to the low or limited quality of life of infants who are chronically and irreversibly comatose, or for whom continued, aggressive treatment would be either "futile" or "inhumane." Continued denial of judgments about the quality of life, on the part of those who have endorsed these plausible exceptions, is either disingenuous or self-deceptive.

Quality-of-life judgments, we believe, can neither be uncritically embraced nor categorically rejected when addressing treatment decisions for seriously ill newborns. As John Arras puts it in his illuminating discussion of the topic in Chapter 6, "The proper question is not 'Should quality of life count?'—of course it should, because it is inescapable—but rather 'Which quality of life position should we adopt?' " To this end, Arras's distinction between *comparative* and *noncomparative* judgments is extremely useful. The former compare the value of an infant's life with some standard or norm based on a life without disability or serious illness. The latter focus exclusively on the condition of the infant and the question of the likely effects on the infant itself of one or another proposed medical intervention. Rejection of comparative quality-of-life judgments, Arras points out, does not require rejection of noncomparative judgments. And acceptance of noncomparative judgments does not, in itself, license or justify comparative judgments. Wholesale advocacy and wholesale condemnation should, as Arras puts it, now give way to "an honest, open, and carefully nuanced debate about the *limits* of quality of life reasoning."

Family and Society

If the moral status of the infant is the same as that of the adult and if noncomparative as well as comparative judgments of the quality of life are impermissible, all lives will have to be sustained for as long as possible. The fact that few who are required to *defend* (rather than simply propound) a position on this matter are likely to maintain such an extreme conclusion suggests that it cannot be thoughtfully upheld. As the three exceptions to the 1985 final rule governing the withholding of treatment from disabled infants tacitly admit, no simple appeal to the "sanctity of life" can adequately account for the relevant complexities. Other features of the situation must also be taken into account. The question now is whether these should ever include the burdens, on family and society, of raising and providing for seriously impaired infants and the children and adults they will become.

Although in the not-too-distant past some thoughtful physicians regarded such burdens as relevant to decision making (30, 31), this view is now out of official favor, at least in the United States. The prevailing outlook is, perhaps, best expressed by the President's Commission for the Study of Ethical Problems in Medicine and Biomedical Research in its recommendation that the sole standard for making decisions of this kind should be "the best interests of the infant." "This is a very strict standard," the Commission points out, "in that it excludes consideration of the negative effects of an impaired child's life on other persons, including parents, siblings, and society" (32: p. 219). But can these "negative effects" always be excluded from responsible decision making?

Consider first the family. Although there are cases where raising a disabled infant brings out the best of and strengthens an entire family, we must resist the temptation to base overall policy on an unbalanced diet of success stories. In other cases, where the marital bonds may be more vulnerable, where the needs of other children cannot be ignored, where personal temperament, social and economic factors, and so on are not so favorable, the presence of a seriously disabled child has resulted in increased levels of divorce, emotional disturbance in parents and siblings, and various levels of child abuse and neglect (33, 34). Not everyone, it turns out, has the personal makeup or favorable circumstances for raising a seriously impaired child. If, then, we endorse the restrictive guidelines of the federal government or the "very strict standard" recommended by the President's Commission, we must, if we are to act in good faith, also do what we can to increase significantly the level of social, psychological, and economic support for the parents of seriously impaired children. We should also try to reduce the barriers to, and stigma of, giving up such children for adoption or foster placement.

This may, however, concede too much to the prevailing outlook. As Carson Strong points out in Chapter 7, there may be cases where the interests of the family should be permitted to take priority over those of the patient, "provided the encroachment of the patient's interests is relatively small and the harm to the family thereby prevented is great." As an example, Strong cites a case where futile life-sustaining treatment of a premature infant was continued for a few days in order to give the family, which was having a difficult time accepting the fact that the baby was dying, a bit more time to adjust. "Although this approach might prolong discomfort for the infant," Strong writes, "it would help prevent serious harm to the family associated with the shock of learning that their daughter's treatment was being terminated. In spite of this slight compromise of the patient's interests, a delay for the family's sake appeared to be the right approach." Whether, and if so to what extent, this approach would be applicable to decisions to withdraw rather than continue life-sustaining treatment will depend on one's view of the extent to which infants have an interest in continued existence. If, for example, one believes that an infant lacks sufficient self-awareness and sense of the future to have a personal interest in continued life, one may want to place greater weight on the effect of continued aggressive treatment on the interests of the family.

If, however, *society's* interests in the same infant's continued existence are taken into consideration, they might be sufficient to override contrary interests of the family. Yet a society's interests in the lives of disabled infants must extend beyond the intensive care unit. How much social, psychological, and economic support is society prepared to provide for impaired children and their families? How many of us are prepared to adopt disabled children whose parents find themselves unable to cope with them? And if social, psychological, and economic support is insufficient to provide natural, foster, or adoptive parents for all such children or if certain infants cannot be adequately taken care of in the home, are we willing as a society to pay the bill for *decent* institutional care? "Handicapped infants salvaged in neonatal care units," Angell observed, "grow into handicapped children who often require more care and support than their families can provide. The numbers of these children are growing as the technology to save them improves. What happens to them?" (35: p. 660). A recent examination of pediatric nursing homes suggests that, "Low standards of care and financial disincentives have resulted in less than optimal educational and rehabilitative services [for children with multiple severe handicaps for whom care in the community was unrealistic]" (36: p. 640). A society's expressed interest in an infant's continued life, we believe, must be matched, in dollars, with a concern with its life as a child and an adult and with a concern for the family as a whole. To disregard the latter is to weaken considerably whatever moral claim we might have to override parental decisions having to do with the former.

Although we have discussed them separately, it is important to bear in mind that questions about the moral status of the infant, the quality of life, and the decision-making authority of family and society are closely interrelated. A position on any one of them is bound to presuppose or have implications for positions on the other two.

Public Policy

Many ethical conflicts are not, at least at present, rationally reconcilable. That is, there is no single theory or set of principles that all persons, insofar as they are rational, ought to embrace and that yields clear, determinate solutions to all, or perhaps even most, of the ethical issues we have identified. In what follows we will briefly explain why this is so. Then we will turn to the question of devising policy on matters of rationally irreconcilable moral conflict. Can parties to a deep and rationally irreconcilable conflict in perinatal ethics accept a compromise at the level of policy without compromising their integrity? After briefly characterizing what we will call "integrity-preserving compromise," we suggest that in some cases they can. Parties to various disputes, as well as those charged with developing public policy, should, therefore, develop a deeper understanding of compromise in ethics and the extent to which it can be integrity-preserving.

Rationally Irreconcilable Conflict

Stuart Hampshire has recently compared efforts to reduce all ethical conflict to matters of abstract impersonal reason with the project of Esperanto, the attempt to devise a comprehensive, universal language. The latter does not succeed, Hampshire suggests, because it cannot account for the local and particular circumstances and history that give shape and meaning to our lives: "A language distinguishes a particular people with a particular shared history and with a particular set of shared associations and with largely unconscious memories, preserved in the metaphors that are imbedded in the vocabulary" (37: p. 135). The same is true, he adds, with some parts of morality, especially those that govern sexual and family relationships and matters of life and death. To restrict the discussion of conflicts involving these aspects of morality to abstract, universal reason is to be as remote and detached from what actually matters to people as is the project of Esperanto. Conflicts about the structure and nature of the family or the moral status of the embryo, fetus, or newborn turn on values and principles, ways of life and world views, that are historically conditioned, contingent, and not fully determined by abstract, universal principles.

Contrary to what many of us would like to believe, the values governing our convictions on such matters are more closely related to sentiment and personal circumstance than to abstract, impersonal reason. They are bound up with particular world views that are themselves rooted in divergent personal, cultural, and historical ways of life. As such, they will often conflict. The world view and way of life of, say, a housewife and mother of five with strong fundamentalist convictions is likely to differ considerably from that of a single, female executive who wants to become a mother through AID, but who has little or no inclination to be married. We can reasonably assume, for example, that they would have differing ethical views on the use of new reproductive technologies or abortion (13). Moreover, advances in science and technology are as likely to create as to ameliorate such differences. "[W]e know," Hampshire writes, "that accelerating natural science and technology often produces effects that are morally ambiguous and uncertain and that they import drastic changes into cherished and admired ways of life" (37: p. 155). Thus as some advances in scientific understanding reduce differences based on ignorance and superstition, other forms of scientific and technological innovation and intervention multiply possibilities and create new ways of differing. Consider, in this connection, the way numerous advances in perinatal medicine have, by providing for the possibility of new or significantly modified ways of life, created new ethical conflicts.

Those who, like Hampshire, emphasize the limits of abstract, universal reason in ethics do not deny that general principles of, say, justice (construed here as including considerations of rights and equality) or utility are at some level applicable to everyone. But, such principles, they maintain, do not fully determine all of our ethical decisions. General principles of justice or utility are, to be sure, capable of showing that murder, rape, slavery, racism, Naziism, sexism and certain other acts and practices are universally wrong. But many actual conflicts, both within and between certain ways of life, cannot be resolved by considerations of justice or utility alone. Such general considerations fail to determine the whole of morality; they do not, to adapt a phrase from Bernard Williams, "go all the way down" (38: p. 108). They do not, for example, go all the way down to the level of particular disputes about surrogate motherhood, the moral status of the embryo, fetus, or newborn, forced cesareans, and so on. Such disputes are rooted in opposing world views (including religious and metaphysical beliefs) and ways of life that do not straightforwardly violate general principles of justice or utility.

Attempts to resolve these matters in terms of one or another general principle will either be controversial or vacuous. Close examination of the frequently labored attempts to provide a concrete, more or less purely utilitarian or Kantian "solution" to these issues will reveal a number of question-begging factual and metaphysical assumptions. The reasoning will incorporate an unacknowledged bias toward one or another world view and way of life. As a result, the practical conclusions will be unacceptable to those who do not share the relevant world view and way of life. It is not, as the proponents of such arguments often suggest, that those who disagree with them are "irrational," but rather that what is at stake involves more than abstract, impersonal reason. Philosophical arguments that avoid commitment to one or another world view and way of life may avoid such biases, but they pay a heavy price for their neutrality; they are usually so abstract and "theoretical" as to have no practical bearing on the issue at hand. As Hilary Putnam has wryly observed, "When a philosopher 'solves' an ethical problem for one, one feels as if one had asked for a subway token and been given a passenger ticket valid for the first interplanetary passenger-carrying spaceship instead" (39: p. 3).

A more forthright justification of a particular ethical position on a controversial matter in perinatal ethics would acknowledge that it is rooted in a certain world view that gives shape and meaning to a certain way of life and that this is a legitimate, perhaps superior, way of life that does not violate universal principles of justice or utility. In giving such a justification, one would be trying to persuade others of the validity of this world view and way of life and urging that they either adopt it themselves or modify their own views so as to approximate it more closely. But as for oneself, at least initially, "there is no choice." To abandon one's position on this issue, one thinks at the outset, would be to compromise one's identity and integrity as a particular person. Ethical theorists who dismiss this type of justification—who disregard the importance of culturally and historically conditioned sentiment and the importance of identity, integrity, and a person's world view and way of life—underestimate the extent to which many of the things that really matter to us, that give shape and meaning to our lives, are grounded in what is local and particular rather than universal and general.

In Chapter 8 Robert A. Hahn reveals the diversity of world views and ways of life with regard to perinatal matters among four North American ethnic groups (Navajo, Chinese, lower class blacks, and middle-class whites) and members of one medical speciality (obstetrics). In so doing he provides a number of concrete examples of diverse and occasionally conflicting world views and ways of life having to do with perinatal concerns. "The fact of these differences," as Hahn puts it, "and some of the specific differences themselves, carry profound implications for the development of . . . perinatal ethics." It is, for example, most unlikely that mutually satisfactory resolutions of conflicts about such matters as the moral status of the embryo, fetus, or newborn can be based on abstract, universal reason alone. Solutions of this kind will require widespread agreement on a single world view and way of life for all. History gives us little reason to believe that such a dream (others might plausibly characterize it as a *nightmare*) will soon come true. What Isaiah Berlin has said about human conflict in general seems, therefore, to be especially applicable to ethical issues at the outset of life:

[T]he belief that some single formula can in principle be found whereby all the diverse ends of men can be harmoniously realized is demonstrably false. . . . [T]he ends of men are many, and not all of them are in principle compatible with each other . . . [thus] the possibility of conflict—and of tragedy—can never be wholly eliminated from human life, either personal or social. The necessity of choosing between absolute claims is an inescapable characteristic of the human condition (40: p. 164).

Compromise

Although many ethical conflicts do not admit of rational *resolution*, reason can nonetheless play an important role in adjudicating or ameliorating them. While unable to resolve disagreements rooted in opposing and incommensurable world views and ways of life, philosophical reason may, in at least some cases, contribute to the development of a sound, mutually acceptable compromise.

A compromise, as understood here, is a position that more or less "splits the difference" between two opposing positions and that is arrived at through a process of give-and-take discussion involving mutual respect and mutual concession. The term 'compromise' refers both to an *outcome* and to a *process*; as outcome it is *something reached*, and as process, *a way of reaching*.

A compromise position, we must also note, is importantly different from a middle-of-the-road or synthesis position. If, for example, two parties holding conflicting positions A and B, respectively, each comes to regard a third position S (a synthesis that combines the strongest features of A and B while avoiding their drawbacks) as superior to each A and B and then embrace it, we do not have a compromise. There has been no compromise or concession by either party. In adopting S each has abandoned what is now regarded as a less correct view (either A or B) for one (S) that is, on its own terms, much better. The result is one form of (rational) *resolution* of the initial conflict, not a compromise.

Now, however, suppose that the party holding A and the party holding B remain wedded to their respective positions but find themselves in circumstances requiring a nondeferrable, joint decision on the matter. Mutually respectful give-and-take discussion leads them to acknowledge the historical roots and contingency of their respective positions (that is, that the positions are rooted in opposing world views and ways of life) and to recognize various degrees of factual uncertainty, moral complexity, and the desirability of maintaining a continuing, cooperative relationship (they are, in some sense, "stuck with each other"). If continued efforts to persuade each other of the superiority of their respective views are unsuccessful, they may then agree to a compromise position, C, which seems somehow to split the difference between A and B. Each party will, in this event, make certain concessions to the other for the sake of agreement on a single course of action that seems to have some independent validity and to capture as much as the spirit of A as it does of B, and vice versa. The matter is not, however, fully settled; there is no closure, no final harmony. A compromise is not, as we understand it here, a rational resolution. It makes the best of what both parties to the disagreement regard as a bad situation; and each may continue to do what it can to persuade the other (or some third party to whom each is trying to appeal) of the superiority of either A or B or to see that the same situation does not arise in the future.

As an example of a compromise of this sort, consider the Warnock Committee's recommendation on the question of research using human embryos (9). Moral opinion on this matter was (and still is) deeply divided. At the root of the controversy are opposing views of the moral status of the embryo. Those who regard the embryo as having the same status as an adult human being are strongly opposed to any research of this kind. Those who regard the moral status of the human embryo as considerably less than that of an adult are heavily influenced by the undeniable utilitarian advantages of such research. The Warnock Committee was charged with making a recommendation at the level of national policy on this deep and highly charged question. Although moral views on this matter were divided, a policy embodied in law would necessarily be singular and binding on all. Moreover the question could no longer be deferred. Legislation was needed on the matter, and soon.

The most basic recommendation (of the majority of the Committee's members) on the question of research using human embryos—namely that such research would be permitted, subject to certain restrictions, only up to 14 days from fertilization and unconditionally forbidden thereafter—seems to have been a compromise between the two polar positions found in society. As Warnock has put it, "In the end the Inquiry felt bound to argue, *partly* on Utilitarian grounds, that the benefits that had come in the past from research using human embryos were so great (and were likely to be even greater in the future), that such research had to be permitted; but that it should be permitted only at the very earliest stage of the development of the embryo" (41: p. 517). Each polar position to the disagreement (that representing an extreme conservative view of the moral standing of the embryo and that representing a considerably more liberal view) received part, but not all, of what it was after.

Mary Warnock herself, however, does not quite see it in this way. She notes that the Committee's recommendations may be disappointing to Ministers of Parliament who, understandably enough, may have been hoping for "a solution to a problem essentially insoluble."

In the case of our Committee, for example, it was hoped, I now see, that the cool and reasonable voice of philosophy would reconcile the irreconcilable and find a compromise where none can exist. There may even have been a secret belief that there is a right solution which could be proved right, if it were only found. But Ministers, like the rest of humanity, have to realize that in matters of morality this is not possible. Society may value things, genuinely and quite properly, which are incompatible with each other (9: p. 99).

We can agree with everything in this passage except the way Warnock uses the term "compromise." What she means by "compromise" we would label a "rational resolution" or "synthesis." It is because, as she points out, neither a rational resolution nor a synthesis of the opposing views on, say, the question of the moral status of the embryo was possible, that her Committee had to settle for what we call a "compromise."

That the Committee's final recommendation on this matter was, indeed, what we have labeled a compromise is reinforced by Thomas H. Murray in Chapter 9 when he points out that no single theory of the moral status of the human embryo can embrace, without contradiction, all of the Committee's recommendations. But, he adds, "the Committee did not need to provide a final, authoritative answer to this question. Its task was to find a compromise that would permit important social needs to be fulfilled, without outraging widely and deeply held moral values." Similar forms of compromise, Murray suggests, are embodied in plausible social policy recommendations addressing other issues in perinatal ethics, including the moral status of the fetus, the moral status of the newborn, the legitimacy of judgments about the quality of life, and the extent to which interests other than those of the newborn ought to be taken into account in making decisions.

Integrity

In addition to the use we have emphasized, the term "compromise" also has a well-known pejorative use. Talk of *compromising one's principles* or *compromising one's integrity* suggests that compromise is ethically dishonorable—a sign of moral weakness, hypocrisy, opportunism, and so on. Some go as far as to say that a person cannot embrace a compromise position on a matter of ethical importance without compromising (in the sense of *betraying*) his or her basic ethical convictions (42). But is this always so? Is it possible to hold a particular position, say either *A* or *B*, on a particular issue in perinatal ethics, and at the same time agree on matters of policy affecting all to a certain compromise position, C, without compromising one's integrity? We think it is.

To see how a compromise of this sort may be integrity-preserving it is important, following a suggestion of Arthur Kuflik, to distinguish 1) what one believes ought to be done in a particular (kind of) case, leaving aside for the moment that there is a rationally irreconcilable conflict, from 2) what one judges ought to be done *all things considered* when among the things to be considered are that there is such a conflict and that a single decision affecting all of the contending parties must soon be made:

> When an issue is in dispute there is more to be considered than the issue itself—for example, the importance of peace, the presumption against settling matters by force, the intrinsic good in participating in a process in which each side must hear the other side out and try to see matters from the other's point of view, the extent to which the matter does admit reasonable differences of opinion and the significance of a settlement in which each party feels assured of the other's respect for its own seriousness and sincerity in the matter (43: p. 51).

These considerations of tolerance and mutual respect reflect values and principles that many of us hold dear and that partially determine who we are and what we stand for. If, therefore, those who disagree with us on a particular issue in perinatal ethics also place a high value on toleration and mutual respect, agreeing to a plausible compromise may threaten the integrity of neither party. On the contrary, taking into consideration *all* of our values and principles, together with the fact that we disagree and our disagreement is rationally irreconcilable, the compromise position may be more integrity-preserving than any available alternative.

The main point is that, as most of us will on reflection acknowledge, our identity is constituted in part by a complex constellation of occasionally conflicting values and principles. In certain cases it will not be possible to act in accord with all of them. We may, for example, believe both in a polar position (for example, *A* or *B*) on an issue in perinatal ethics *and* in the values identified in the foregoing passage from Kuflik. In such cases of *internal* as well as external conflict we will often pursue that course of action that seems, on balance, to follow from the preponderance of our central and most highly cherished and rationally defensible values and principles. "Where ultimate values are irreconcilable," Berlin has written, "clear-cut solutions cannot, in principle, be found. To decide rationally in such situations is to decide in the light of general ideals, the over-all pattern of life pursued by a man or a group or a society" (40: p. l). If, as we suppose, the overall "pattern of life" favored by most of us and the groups to which we belong and our society is (or should be) one that includes a high degree of trying to see matters from the other's point of view, an understanding of the extent to which certain disagreements are rationally irreconcilable, a presumption against settling matters by rank or force, and so on, it would not be surprising if a compromise on, say, a matter of hospital or social policy with regard to a strongly contested issue in perinatal ethics, were occasionally to be more integrity-preserving than the imposition of either of the polar alternatives.

We have already suggested that the Warnock Committee's recommendation on embryo research amounts to a compromise. Others have characterized the final version of the federal government's "Baby Doe" regulations as a compromise as well (44). Some have also recommended compromise in general and particular forms of compromise as the best way to address the festering problem of abortion in American social and political life (45, 46). However, not all who are generally sympathetic to compromise are optimistic about its applicability to abortion. Kristen Luker, for example, predicts that

the abortion debate is likely to remain bitter and divisive for years to come. Beliefs about the rightness or wrongness of abortion both represent and illuminate our more cherished beliefs about the world, about motherhood, and about what it means to be human. It should not surprise us that these views admit of very little compromise (13: p. 10).

In this she may prove to be correct.

There are, we admit, important limitations to compromise. It is not, for example, value-neutral. Indeed, an emphasis on the ethical and practical benefits of compromise, as Robert A. Hahn suggests at the end of Chapter 8, is part of a distinctive world view and way of life; one that explicitly recognizes a plurality of divergent and occasionally conflicting values and principles. It assumes an "anthropological perspective" and places a premium on understanding opposing viewpoints and positions, mutual respect, dialogue, weighing the consequences of our actions on others, and so on. This is not everyone's perspective, nor is there an entirely neutral, abstract philosophical argument to show that it should be (47, 48). It is, however, a perspective that is presupposed by many of our democratic traditions and that recommends itself on pragmatic grounds to policymakers in an avowedly pluralistic society. It is also reinforced by various contributors to this book.

Ethical issues at the outset of life are frequently grounded in conflicting world views and ways of life. They involve moral complexity, factual and metaphysical uncertainty, continuing cooperative relationships (among health professionals, patients, families, and society), and impending, nondeferrable decisions. A deeper understanding of the nature of the issues and the limits of abstract, impersonal reason will, we believe, lead to greater appreciation of compromise and the extent to which it can be integrity-preserving.

Conclusion

There are no easy answers to the ethical issues identified and discussed in the chapters that follow. Our overriding aim is not so much to dispense authoritative conclusions as to deepen the reader's understanding and to enable him or her to participate more effectively in the ongoing discussions and debates. In some cases informed and mutually respectful discussion and debate about these matters will eventually result in well-grounded, rational resolutions. This, for example, is what seems to have happened during the past 20 years with regard to the issue of "brain death" (49). In other cases such resolutions will remain elusive. But even here, a more sophisticated understanding of the depth and complexity of the issues will often convince the opposing parties that those holding different views are not callous, irrational, or otherwise "ethically defective." In cases requiring joint action or a single policy, such understanding may be the first step toward the development of a mutually satisfying compromise. And on matters as complex and divisive as these, such a result, though falling short of closure and final harmony, is a significant advance.

References

1. Walters W. Ethical aspects of transexualism and its managements. Bioethics News (Monash U) 1984;4(1):13–20.
2. Annas G. Redefining parenthood and protecting embryos: why we need new laws. Hastings Cent Rep 1984;14(5):50–52.
3. Somerville MA. Birth technology, parenting and "deviance." Int J Law Psych 1982;5:123–153.
4. Strong C, Schinfeld JS. The single woman and artificial insemination by donor. J Reprod Med 1984;29(5):293–299.
5. McGuire M, Alexander NJ. Artificial insemination of single women. Fertility Sterility 1985;43(2):182–183.
6. Childress JF. Appeals to conscience. Ethics 1979;89:316–321.
7. Curie-Cohen M, Luttrel L, Shapiro S. Current practice of artificial insemination by donor in the United States. N Engl J Med 1979;300:585.
8. Kuhse H, Singer P. Should the baby live? Oxford: Oxford U Press, 1985.
9. Warnock M. A question of life. Oxford: Basil Blackwell, 1985.

10. Callahan D. How technology is changing the abortion debate. Hastings Cent Rep 1986;16:33–42.
11. Brambati B, Simoni G, Fabro, S, eds. Fetal diagnosis during the first trimester. New York: Marcel Dekker, 1986.
12. Harris L, et al. Study No 854005. 1985.
13. Luker K. Abortion and the politics of motherhood. Berkeley and Los Angeles: U of California, 1984.
14. Feinberg J. Abortion. In: Regan, T, ed. Matters of life and death, 2d ed. New York: Random House, 1986.
15. Warren MA. On the moral and legal status of abortion. Monist 1973;57:43–61. Reprinted with postscript (1982) in: Feinberg J, ed. The problem of abortion, 2d ed. Belmont, CA: Wadsworth, 1984.
16. Singer P. Practical ethics. Cambridge, England: Cambridge U Press, 1979.
17. Tooley M. Abortion and infanticide. Oxford: Oxford U Press, 1983.
18. Noonan JT. An almost absolute value in history. In: Noonan JT, ed. The morality of abortion: legal and historical perspectives. Cambridge, MA: MIT Press, 1970.
19. Sumner LW. A third way. In: Feinberg J, ed. The problem of abortion, 2d ed. Belmont, CA: Wadsworth, 1984.
20. Mackenzie TB, Nagel TC, Rothman BK. When a pregnant woman endangers her fetus. Hastings Cent Rep 1986;16:24–25.
21. Grannum PA, Copel JA, Plaxe SC, Sciosa AL, Hobbins JC. In utero exchange transfusion by direct intravascular injection in severe erythroblastosio fetalis. N Engl J Med 1986;314:1431–1434.
22. Annas GJ. Forced cesareans: the most unkindest cut of all. Hastings Cent Rep 1982;12:16–17,45.
23. Federal Register 1985;50:14873–14892.
24. Moskop JC, Saldanha RL. The Baby Doe rule: still a threat. Hastings Cent Rep 1986;16:8–14.
25. Weil WB Jr. The Baby Doe regulations: another view of change. Hastings Cent Rep 1986;16:12–13.
26. Brock D. Life-support decisions for newborns. QQ—Rep Center for Philosophy and Public Policy 1985;4:12–14.
27. Robertson JA. Involuntary euthanasia of defective newborns: a legal analysis. Stanford Law Rev 1975;27:213–256.
28. Murray TH. The final anticlimactic rule on Baby Doe. Hastings Cent Rep 1985;15:5–9.
29. Benjamin M. The infant's interest in continued life: a sentimental fiction. Bioethics Rep 1983;5–7.
30. Duff RS, Campbell AGM. Moral and ethical dilemmas in the special-care nursery. N Engl J Med 1973;289:890–894.
31. Duff RS, Campbell AGM. On deciding the care of severely handicapped or dying persons: with particular reference to infants. Pediatrics 1976;57:487–493.
32. President's Commission for the Study of Ethical Problems in Medicine and Biomedical and Behavioral Research. Deciding to forgo life-sustaining treatment. Washington, DC: U.S. Government Printing Office, 1983.
33. Tew B, Payne EH, Lawrence KM. Must a family with a handicapped child be a handicapped family? Dev Med Child Neurol 1974;16:95–98.

34. Kew S. Handicap and family crisis. London: Pitman, 1975.
35. Angell M. Handicapped children: Baby Doe and Uncle Sam. N Engl J of Med 1983;309:659–661.
36. Glick PS, et al. Pediatric nursing homes. N Engl J Med 1983;309:640–646.
37. Hampshire S. Morality and conflict. Cambridge, MA: Harvard U Press, 1983.
38. Williams B. Ethics and the limits of philosophy. Cambridge, MA: Harvard U Press, 1985.
39. Putnam H. How not to solve ethical problems: the Lindley Lecture. Lawrence, KA: Department of Philosophy–U of Kansas, 1983.
40. Berlin I. Four essays on liberty. Oxford: Oxford U Press, 1969.
41. Warnock M. Moral thinking and government policy: the Warnock Committee on human embryology. Millbank Mem Fund Quart 1985;63:504–521.
42. Rand A. The virtue of selfishness. New York: Signet, 1964.
43. Kuflik A. Morality and compromise. In: Pennock RJ, Chapman JW, eds. Compromise in ethics, law, and politics. New York: New York U Press, 1979.
44. Kerr K. Negotiating the compromises. Hastings Cent Rep 1985;15:6–7.
45. Sher G. Subsidized abortion: moral rights and moral compromise. Philosophy Public Affairs 1981;10:361–372.
46. Frohock F. Abortion: a case study in law and morals. Westport CT: Greenwood, 1983.
47. Rorty R. Philosophy and the mirror of nature. Princeton NJ: Princeton U Press, 1979.
48. Rorty R. Consequences of pragmatism. Minneapolis: U of Minnesota Press, 1982.
49. President's Commission for the Study of Ethical Problems in Medicine and Biomedical and Behavioral Research. Defining death. Washington, DC: U.S. Government Printing Office, 1981.

II

Preimplantation Period

2

Creating Embryos*

PETER SINGER

The treatment of human embryos became a matter of public controversy in July 1978. That month saw the birth of Louise Brown, the first human being to have developed from an embryo which at some point in its existence was outside a human body. This marked the beginning of what can properly be called a revolution in human reproduction. The point is not that *in vitro* fertilization (the technique used to make possible the birth of Louise Brown) is itself so extraordinary. On the contrary, *in vitro* fertilization, or IVF, can be seen as simply a way of overcoming certain forms of infertility, such as blocked fallopian tubes. In this sense, IVF is no more revolutionary than a microsurgical operation to remove the blockage in the tubes. But IVF is revolutionary because it brings the embryo out of the human body. Once the embryo is in the open, human beings can observe it, manipulate it, and make life-or-death decisions about it. These possibilities make IVF, and its future applications, a subject of the utmost moral importance.

Consider what has already happened, all within the first decade after Brown. Women who do not produce eggs have been given eggs by other women who do; they have then given birth to babies to whom they are genetically entirely unrelated (1).

Embryos have been frozen in liquid nitrogen, stored for more than a year, thawed, and then transferred to women who have given birth to normal children. In one case, two "twins"—that is, children conceived from eggs produced by a single ovulatory cycle—were born 16 months apart. Another case illustrated the pitfalls of embryo freezing: two embryos, in storage in a Melbourne laboratory, were orphaned when their parents were killed in a plane crash, apparently leaving no instructions regarding the disposition of their embryos (1).

Scientists have begun to speculate on the medical purposes to which embryos might be put. Dr. Robert Edwards, the scientist who, together with Patrick Steptoe, made it possible for Louise Brown to be born, has suggested that if embryos could be grown for about 17 days, we could

---

* *This chapter is based on work done together with Deane Wells and was previously published in* (1).

take from them developing blood cells which would have the potential to overcome such fatal diseases as sickle cell anemia and perhaps leukemia (2).

There was a time when our ethical codes could slowly adapt to changing circumstances. Those days are gone. We have to decide, right now, whether the moral status of embryos is such that it is wrong to freeze them or experiment upon them. We have also to make an immediate decision on whether there is any objection to allowing some women to carry and bring to birth embryos to which they have no genetic link. We have, at most, until the end of the century to decide how to handle new technologies for selecting and manipulating embryos, technologies that will force us to ask which human qualities are most desirable. We must start by acquainting ourselves with the new techniques and deciding which of them should form part of the society in which we live.

IVF: The Simple Case

The so-called simple case of IVF is that in which a married, infertile couple use an egg taken from the wife and sperm taken from the husband, and all embryos created are inserted into the womb of the wife. This case allows us to consider the ethics of IVF in itself, without the complications of the many other issues that can arise in different circumstances. Then we can go on to look at these complications separately.

The Technique

The technique itself is now well known and is fast becoming a routine part of infertility treatment in many countries. The infertile woman is given a hormone treatment to induce her ovaries to produce more than one egg in her next cycle. Her hormone levels are carefully monitored to detect the precise moment at which the eggs are ripening. At this time the eggs are removed. This is usually done by laparoscopy, a minor operation in which a fine tube is inserted into the woman's abdomen and the egg is sucked out up the tube. A laparoscope, a kind of periscope illuminated by fiber optics, is also inserted into the abdomen so that the surgeon can locate the place where the ripe egg is to be found. Instead of laparoscopy, some IVF teams are now using ultrasound techniques, which eliminate the need for a general anesthetic.

Once the eggs have been collected they are placed in culture in small glass dishes known as petri dishes, not in test tubes despite the popular label of "test-tube babies." Sperm is then obtained from the male partner by means of masturbation and placed with the egg. Fertilization follows in at least 80 percent of the ripe eggs. The resulting embryos are allowed to cleave once or twice and are usually transferred to the woman some 48 to 72 hours after fertilization. The actual transfer is done via the vagina and is a simple procedure.

It is after the transfer, when the embryo is back in the uterus and beyond the scrutiny of medical science, that things are most likely to go wrong. Even with the most experienced IVF teams, the majority of embryos transferred fail to implant in the uterus. One pregnancy for every five transfers is currently considered to be a good working average for a competent IVF team. Many of the newer teams fail to achieve anything like this rate. Nevertheless, there are so many units around the world now practicing IVF that thousands of babies have been produced as a result of the technique. IVF has ceased to be experimental and is now a routine, if still "last resort" method of treating some forms of infertility.

Objections to the Simple Case

There is some opposition to IVF even in the simple case. The most frequently heard objections are as follows:
1. IVF is unnatural.
2. IVF is risky for the offspring.
3. IVF separates the procreative and the conjugal aspects of marriage and so damages the marital relationship.
4. IVF is illicit because it involves masturbation.
5. Adoption is a better solution to the problem of childlessness.
6. IVF is an expensive luxury and the resources would be better spent elsewhere.
7. IVF allows increased male control over reproduction and hence threatens the status of women in the community.

We can deal swiftly with the first four of these objections. If we were to reject medical advances on the grounds that they are "unnatural" we would be rejecting modern medicine as a whole, for the very purpose of the medical enterprise is to resist the ravages of nature which would otherwise shorten our lives and make them much less pleasant. If anything is in accordance with the nature of our species, it is the application of our intelligence to overcome adverse situations in which we find ourselves. The application of IVF to infertile couples is a classic example of this application of human intelligence.

The claim that IVF is risky for the offspring is one that was argued with great force before IVF became a widely used technique. It is sufficient to note that the results of IVF so far have happily refuted these fears. The most recent Australian figures, for example, based on 934 births, indicate that the rate of abnormality was 2.7%, which is very close to the national average of 1.5%. When we take into account the greater average age of women seeking IVF, as compared with the child-bearing population as a whole, it does not seem that the *in vitro* technique itself adds to the risk of an abnormal offspring. This view is reinforced by the fact that the abnormalities were all ones that arise with the ordinary method of reproduction; there have been no new "monsters" produced by IVF (3). Perhaps we still cannot claim with statistical certainty that the risk of defect is no higher with IVF than with the more common method of conception; but if the risk is higher at all, it would appear to be only very slightly higher, and still within limits which may be considered acceptable.

The third and fourth objections have been urged by spokesmen for certain religious groups, but they are difficult to defend outside the confines of particular religions. Few infertile couples will take seriously the view that their marital relationship will be damaged if they use the technique which offers them the best chance of having their own child. It is in any case extraordinarily paternalistic for anyone else to tell a couple that they should not use IVF because it will harm their marriage. That, surely, is for them to decide.

The objection to masturbation comes from a similar source and can be even more swiftly dismissed. Religious prohibitions on masturbation are taboos from past times which even religious spokesmen are beginning to consider outdated. Moreover, even if one could defend a prohibition on masturbation for sexual pleasure—perhaps on the (very tenuous) ground that sexual activity is wrong unless it is directed either toward procreation or toward the strengthening of the bond between marriage partners—it would be absurd to extend a prohibition with that kind of rationale to a case in which masturbation is being used in the context of a marriage and precisely in order to make reproduction possible. (The fact that some religions do persist in regarding masturbation as wrong, even in these circumstances, is indicative of the folly of an ethical system based on absolute rules, irrespective of the circumstances in which those rules are being applied, or the consequences of their application.)

Overpopulation and the Allocation of Resources

The next two objections, however, deserve more careful consideration. In an overpopulated world in which there are so many children who cannot be properly fed and cared for, there is something incongruous about using all the ingenuity of modern medicine to create more children. And similarly, when there are so many deaths caused by preventable diseases, is there not something wrong with the priorities which lead us to develop expensive techniques for overcoming the relatively less serious problem of infertility?

These objections are sound to the following extent: in an ideal world we would find loving families for unwanted children before we created additional children; and in an ideal world we would clear up all the preventable ill-health and malnutrition-related diseases before we went on to tackle the problem of infertility. But is it appropriate to ask, of IVF alone, whether it can stand the test of measurement against what we would do in an ideal world? In an ideal world, none of us would consume more than our fair share of resources. We would not drive expensive cars while others die for the lack of drugs costing a few cents. We would not eat a diet rich in wastefully produced animal products while others cannot get enough to nourish their bodies. We cannot demand more of infertile couples than we are ready to demand of ourselves. If fertile couples are free to have large families of their own, rather than adopt destitute children from overseas, infertile couples must also be free to do what they can to have their own families. In both cases, overseas adoption, or perhaps the adoption of local children who are unwanted because of some impairment, should be considered; but if we are not going to make this compulsory in the former case, it should not be made compulsory in the latter.

There is a further question: to what extent do infertile couples have a right to assistance from community medical resources? Again, however, we must not single out IVF for harsher treatment than we give to other medical techniques. If tubal surgery is available and covered by one's health insurance, or is offered as part of a national health scheme, then why should IVF be treated any differently? And if infertile couples can get free or subsidized psychiatry to help them overcome the psychological problems of infertility, there is something absurd about denying them free or subsidized treatment which could overcome the root of the problem, rather than the symptoms. By today's standards, after all, IVF is not an inordinately expensive medical technique; and there is no country, as far as I know, which limits its provision of free or subsidized health care to those cases in which the patient's life is in danger. Once we extend medical care to cover cases of injury, incapacity, and psychological distress, IVF has a strong claim to be included among the range of free or subsidized treatments available.

The Effect on Women

The final objection is one that has come from some feminists. In a recently published collection of essays by women titled *Test-Tube Women: What Future for Motherhood?*, several contributors are suspicious of the

new reproductive technology. None is more hostile than Robyn Rowland, an Australian sociologist, who writes:

Ultimately the new technology will be used for the benefit of men and to the
detriment of women. Although technology itself is not always a negative development, the real question has always been—who controls it? Biological technology is in the hands of men (4).

And Rowland concludes with a warning as dire as any uttered by the
most conservative opponents of IVF:

What may be happening is the last battle in the long war of men against women.
Women's position is most precarious . . . we may find ourselves without a
product of any kind with which to bargain. For the history of "mankind"
women have been seen in terms of their value as child-bearers. We have to ask,
if that last power is taken and controlled by men, what role is envisaged for
women in the new world? Will women become obsolete? Will we be fighting to
retain or reclaim the right to bear children—has patriarchy conned us once
again? I urge you sisters to be vigilant (4).

I can see little basis for such claims. For a start, women have figured
quite prominently in the leading IVF teams in Britain, Australia, and the
United States: Jean Purdy was an early colleague of Edwards and Steptoe in the research that led to the birth of Louise Brown; Linda Mohr has
directed the development of embryo freezing at the Queen Victoria
Medical Centre in Melbourne; and in the United States Georgeanna
Jones and Joyce Vargyas have played leading roles in the groundbreak-
ing clinics in Norfolk, Virginia, and at the University of Southern California, respectively. It seems odd for a feminist to neglect the contributions these women have made.

Even if one were to grant, however, that the technology remains
predominantly in male hands, it has to be remembered that it was developed in response to the needs of infertile couples. From interviews I
have conducted and meetings I have attended, my impression is that
while both partners are often very concerned about their childlessness,
in those cases in which one partner is more distressed than the other by
this situation, that partner is usually the woman. Feminists usually accept that this is so, attributing it to the power of social conditioning in a
patriarchal society; but the origin of the strong female desire for children
is not really what is in question here. The question is: in what sense is
the new technology an instrument of male domination over women? If it
is true that the technology was developed at least as much in response to
the needs of women as in response to the needs of men, then it is hard
to see why a feminist should condemn it.

It might be objected that whatever the origins of IVF and no matter how benign it may be when used to help infertile couples, the further development of techniques such as ectogenesis—the growth of the embryo from conception totally outside the body, in an artificial womb—will reduce the status of women. Again, it is not easy to see why this should be so. Ectogenesis will, if it is ever successful, provide a choice for women. Shulamith Firestone argued several years ago in her influential feminist work *The Dialectic of Sex* (5) that this choice will remove the fundamental biological barrier to complete equality. Hence Firestone welcomed the prospect of ectogenesis and condemned the low priority given by our male-dominated society to research in this area.

Firestone's view is surely more in line with the drive to sexual equality than the position taken by Rowland. If we argue that to break the link between women and childbearing would be to undermine the status of women in our society, what are we saying about the ability of women to obtain true equality in other spheres of life? I am not so pessimistic about the abilities of women to achieve equality with men across the broad range of human endeavor. For that reason I think women will be helped, rather than harmed, by the development of a technology which makes it possible for them to have children without being pregnant. As Nancy Breeze, a very differently inclined contributor to the same collection of essays, puts it:

Two thousand years of morning sickness and stretch marks have not resulted in liberation for women or children. If you should run into a Petri dish, it could turn out to be your best friend. So rock it; don't knock it! (6)

So to sum up this discussion of the ethics of the simple case of IVF: the ethical objections urged against IVF under these conditions are not strong. They should not count against going ahead with IVF when it is the best way of overcoming infertility and when the infertile couple are not prepared to consider adoption as a means of overcoming their problem. There is, admittedly, a serious question about how much of the national health budget should be allocated to this area. But then, there are serious questions about the allocation of resources in other areas of medicine as well.

IVF: Other Cases

IVF can be used in circumstances that differ from those of the simple case in the following respects:
1. The couple may not be legally married; or there may be no couple at all, the patient being a single woman.

2. The couple may not be infertile but may wish to use IVF for some other reason, for instance because the woman carries a genetic defect.
3. The sperm, or the egg, or both, may come from another person, not from the couple themselves.
4. Some of the embryos created may not be inserted into the womb of the wife; instead they may be frozen and stored for later use, or donated to others, or used for research, or simply discarded.

All of these variations on the simple case raise potentially difficult issues. I say "potentially difficult" because in some cases the difficulties arise only once we consider the more extreme instances. For instance, there are no good grounds for discriminating against couples who are not legally married but have a long-standing de facto relationship; on the other hand one would need to consider more carefully whether to allow a single women to make use of IVF. It is true that single fertile women are entirely free to procreate as irresponsibly as they like; yet the doctor who assists an infertile woman to do the same must take some care that the child in whose creation he or she is assisting will grow up in circumstances that are compatible with a good start in life. A single mother may well be able to provide such circumstances, but it is at least appropriate for the doctor to make some inquiries before going ahead.

IVF for fertile couples when the woman carries a serious genetic defect is scarcely problematic; if we would allow artificial insemination when the man has a similar defect, we should also allow IVF when the woman is the carrier. Here too, however, there is a question about how far we should go. What if the defect is a very minor one? What if there is no defect at all, but the woman wants a donor egg from a friend whose intelligence or beauty she considers superior to her own? A California sperm bank is already offering selected women the sperm of Nobel Prize-winning scientists. It is only a matter of time before eggs are offered in the same manner. Nevertheless it seems clear that as long as IVF is in short supply, those who are infertile or who carry a serious genetic defect should have the first claim upon it. (The issue of genetic selection itself will be touched upon in the final section of this chapter.)

The use of donor sperm, eggs, and embryos raises further questions. There is a precedent in the use of donor sperm in artificial insemination. The lesson that has been learned here is that there is a great need for counseling the couple because there may be psychological problems when one parent is not the genetic parent of the child. There is also the question of whether the child is to be told of her or his genetic origins. Many adopted persons now consider that they have a right to full information about their genetic parents. There is a strong case for saying that the same applies to people born as a result of the use of donor sperm or eggs, and that nonidentifying data about the donor should be released to the parents, with a view to the child being informed at a later stage.

The most controversial of these issues is that of the moral status of the embryo; this is the question at stake when we consider whether to create more embryos than we are willing to put back into the womb at one time. Disposing of the embryos, or using them for research purposes, runs counter to the view held by some that the embryo is a human being with the same right to life as any other human being. Even embryo freezing does little to placate those who take this view, since on present indications the chances of a frozen embryo surviving to become a living child are not high. But, religious doctrines apart, is it plausible to hold that the embryo has a right to life? The moral status of the embryo is perhaps the most fundamental of all the moral issues raised by the reproduction revolution. Many people believe it to be an insoluble philosophical problem, one on which we just have to take our stand, more or less arbitrarily, without hope of persuading those of a different view. I believe, on the contrary, that the issue is amenable to rational discussion. To show this, however, we need to examine the arguments in some detail.

The Moral Status of the Embryo

The Standard Argument

The standard argument in favor of attributing a right to life to the embryo goes like this:

Every human being has a right to life.

A human embryo is a human being.

Therefore the embryo has a right to life.

To avoid questions about capital punishment, or killing in self-defense, it can be stipulated that the term "innocent" is assumed whenever we are talking of human beings and their rights.

The standard argument has a standard response. The standard response is to accept the first premise, that all human beings have a right to life, but to deny the second premise, that the human embryo is a human being. This standard response, however, runs into difficulties, because the embryo is clearly a being of some sort, and it can't possibly be of any other species than *Homo sapiens*. So it seems to follow that it must be a human being. Attempts to say that it only becomes a human being at viability, or at birth, are not entirely convincing. Viability is so closely tied to the state of development of neonatal intensive care that it is hardly the kind of thing that can determine when a being gets a right to live. As for birth, those who draw the line there must explain why an infant born premature at 26 weeks should have a right to life, whereas a fetus of 32 weeks, more developed in every respect, should not. Can location relative to the cervix really make so much difference to one's right to life?

Questioning the First Premise

So the standard argument for attributing a right to life to the embryo can withstand the standard response. It is not easy to mount a direct challenge to the claim that the embryo is a human being. What the standard argument cannot withstand, however, is a more critical examination of its first premise: the premise that every human being has a right to life. At first glance, this seems the stronger premise. Do we really want to deny that every (innocent) human being has a right to life? Are we about to condone murder? No wonder it is at the second premise that most of the fire has been directed. But the first premise is surprisingly vulnerable. Its vulnerability becomes apparent as soon as we cease to take "Every human being has a right to life" as some kind of unquestionable moral axiom, and instead inquire into the moral basis for our particular objection to killing human beings.

By "our particular objection to killing human beings" I mean the objection we have to killing human beings, over and above any objections we may have to killing other living beings, such as pigs and cows and dogs and cats, and even trees and lettuces. Why is it that we think killing human beings is so much more serious than killing these other beings?

The obvious answer is that human beings are different from other animals, and the greater seriousness of killing them is a result of these differences. But which of the many differences between humans and other animals justify such a distinction? Again, the obvious response is that the morally relevant differences are those based on our superior mental powers—our self-awareness, our rationality, our moral sense, our autonomy, or some combination of these. They are the kinds of thing, we are inclined to say, which make us "truly human." To be more precise, they are the kinds of thing which make us *persons*.

That the particular objection to killing human beings rests on such qualities is very plausible. To take the most extreme of the differences between living things, consider a person who is enjoying life, is part of a network of relationships with other people, is looking forward to what tomorrow may bring, and freely choosing the course her or his life will take for the years to come. Now think about a lettuce, which, we can safely assume, knows and feels nothing at all. One would have to be quite mad, or morally blind, or warped, not to see that killing the person is far more serious than killing the lettuce.

We shall postpone, for the present, asking just which of the mental qualities make the difference in the moral seriousness between the killing of a person and the killing of a lettuce. For our immediate purposes, all we need to note is that the plausibility of the assertion that human beings have a right to life depends on the fact that human beings generally possess mental qualities which other living beings do not possess. So should we accept the premise that every human being has a right to life? We may do so, but *only* if we bear in mind that by "human being" here we refer to those beings who have the mental qualities that generally distinguish members of our species from members of other species.

Two Senses of 'Human'

If this is the sense in which we can accept the first premise, however, what of the second premise? It is immediately clear that in the sense of the term "human being" which is required to make the first premise acceptable, the second premise is false. The embryo, especially the early embryo, is obviously not a being with the mental qualities which generally distinguish members of our species from members of other species. The early embryo has no brain, no nervous system. It is reasonable to assume that, so far as its mental life goes, it has no more awareness than a lettuce.

It is still true that the human embryo is a member of the species *Homo sapiens*. That is, as we saw, why it is difficult to deny that the human embryo is a human being. But we can now see that this is not the sense of "human being" we need to make the standard argument work. A valid argument cannot equivocate on the meanings of the central terms it uses. If the first premise is true when "human" means "a being with certain mental qualities" and the second premise is true when "human" means "member of the species *Homo sapiens*," the argument is based on a slide between the two meanings and is invalid.

Speciesism

Can the argument be rescued? It obviously cannot be rescued by claiming that the embryo is a being with the requisite mental qualities. That *might* be arguable for some later stage of the development of the embryo or fetus, but it is impossible to make out the claim for the early embryo.

If the second premise cannot be reconciled with the first in this way, can the first perhaps be defended in a form which makes it compatible with the second? Can it be argued that human beings have a right to life, not because of any moral qualities they may possess, but because they—and not pigs, cows, dogs, or lettuces—are members of the species *Homo sapiens?*

This is a desperate move. Those who make it find themselves having to defend the claim that species membership is *in itself* morally relevant to the wrongness of killing a being. But why should species membership in itself be morally crucial? If we are considering whether it is wrong to destroy something, surely we must look at its actual characteristics, not just the species to which it belongs. If ET and similar visitors from other planets turn out to be sensitive, thinking, planning beings, who get homesick just like we do, would it be acceptable to kill them simply because they are not members of our species? Should you be in any doubt, ask yourself the same kind of question, but with "race" substituted for "species." If we reject the claim that membership of a particular race is *in itself* morally relevant to the wrongness of killing a being, it is not easy to see how we could accept the same claim when based on species membership. Remember that the fact that other races, like our own, can feel, think, and plan for the future is not relevant to this question, for we are considering the simple fact of membership of the particular group—whether race or species—as the *sole* basis for distinguishing between the wrongness of killing those who belong to *our* group, and those who are of some *other* group. As long as we keep this in mind, I am sure that we will conclude that neither race nor species can, *in itself*, provide any justifiable basis for such a distinction.

So the standard argument fails. It fails not because of the standard response that the embryo is not a human being, but because the sense in which the embryo is a human being is not the sense in which we should accept that every human being has a right to life.

The Argument from Potential

At this point in the discussion, those who wish to defend the embryo's right to life often switch ground. We should not, they say, base our views of the status of the embryo on the mental qualities it *actually has while an embryo;* we must, rather, consider what it has the potential to *become.*

Indeed, we do need to consider the moral relevance of the embryo's potential. But this argument is not as easy to grasp as it may appear. If we attempt to set it out in an argument of standard form, as we did with the previous argument, we get

Every potential human being has a right to life.

The embryo is a potential human being.

Therefore the embryo has a right to life.

There is no equivocation in this argument, and its second premise is undoubtedly true. The problem is with the first premise. The claim that every potential human being has a right to life is by no means self-evidently true. We would need to be given good grounds for accepting it. What grounds could there be?

One might try to argue that since full-fledged human beings (those with at least some of the mental qualities I have been discussing) have a right to life, anything with the potential to become a full-fledged human being must also have a right to life. But there is no general rule that a potential X has the rights of an X. If there were, Prince Charles, who is a potential King of England, would now have the rights of a King of England. But he does not.

Another possible argument might go like this: there is nothing of greater moral significance than a thinking, choosing rational being. We value such beings above almost everything else. Therefore anything which can give rise to such a being has value because of what it can become.

What is this argument asserting? It suggests that the destruction of an embryo is wrong because it means that a person who might have existed will now not exist; and since we value people, the destruction of the embryo has caused us to lose something of value. But this proves too much. For destroying an embryo is not the only way of ensuring that a person who might have existed will not exist. If a couple decide, after their second, or third, or fourth child, that their family is complete, it is also the case that a person who might have existed—in fact, several people who might have existed—will not exist. Since some people who oppose abortion also oppose the use of contraceptives, it is worth pointing out that this is true whether the couple use contraceptives, or simply abstain from sexual intercourse during the woman's fertile periods (though admittedly the latter method gives the possible people a greater chance of existence). Yet those who condemn the destruction of embryos do not condemn with equal weight the use of contraceptives, and they generally do not condemn at all the use of sexual abstinence to limit the size of one's family. So it seems that the basis for their objection to the destruction of the embryo cannot be that a person who might have existed will now not exist.

Another example, more relevant to the question of embryo research, suggests the same conclusion. Suppose that a scientist has obtained two ripe eggs from two women, let us call them Jan and Maria. They are hoping to have their eggs fertilized with their husbands' sperm and transferred to their wombs. Jan had her laparoscopy first, her egg was put into a petri dish, and her husband's sperm added to it some hours ago. On checking it, the scientist finds that fertilization has taken place. In the case of Maria's egg the sperm has only just been added to the dish, so fertilization cannot yet have taken place, but the laboratory has a 90 percent success rate for achieving fertilization in these circum-stances, and the scientist is reasonably confident that fertilization will take place within the next few hours. Some would say that to destroy Jan's embryo would be gravely wrong, but to destroy the egg and sperm from Maria and her husband would not be wrong at all, or would be much less seriously wrong. In terms of preventing a possible person from existing, however, the difference is only that there is a slightly higher probability of a person resulting from what is in Jan's petri dish than there is of a person resulting from what is in Maria's petri dish. If the difference in the wrongness of disposing of the contents of the two dishes is greater than this slightly higher probability would justify, it cannot be preventing the existence of a possible future person that makes such disposal wrong. To borrow a phrase from the Oxford philos-opher Jonathan Glover, if it is cake we are after, it doesn't make much difference whether we throw away the ingredients separately, or after they are mixed together (7).

Uniqueness

At this point some will say that it is wrong to destroy an embryo because the embryo already contains the unique genetic basis for a particular person. When a couple abstain from intercourse, or the scientist washes out the petri dish before fertilization has taken place, the genetic consti-tution of the person who might have existed has yet to be determined. This is true, of course, but does it matter? *All* human beings are geneti-cally determinate, and all, except identical siblings, are genetically unique. Imagine that instead of just dropping lots of sperm into a petri dish containing a ripe egg, we carried out a program of artificial repro-duction by singling out just *one* sperm and placing it with the egg. Then, once the sperm had been singled out and placed with the egg, the genetic constitution of the person who could develop from the egg-and-sperm would also have been uniquely determined. Suppose now that after the egg and sperm have been placed together, but before fertilization has taken place, the woman is found to have a medical condition which makes pregnancy inadvisable. Freezing is not available, and there are no patients interested in a donated embryo. Would it be wrong to throw out the egg and sperm at this stage? If you do not think that it would be wrong to dispose of the egg and the sperm in *this* situation (and worse than it would be if the usual procedure, involving millions of sperm, had been used) then you cannot be attributing much moral significance to the existence of a genetically unique entity.

I have pursued the will-o-wisp of potential for a long time—not just today, but over the past five years in which I have been working on this topic. I can understand the view that fertilization is one step in the development of a person and that if potentiality is a matter of degree, the embryo is a degree closer to being a person than a collection of egg and sperm in a petri dish before fertilization has taken place. What I still cannot find is any basis for the view that this difference of degree makes an enormous difference in the moral status of what we have before us.

A Positive Approach

We have now seen the inadequacy of attempts to argue that the early embryo has a right to life. It remains only to say something positive about when in its development the embryo may acquire rights.

The answer must depend on the actual characteristics of the embryo. The minimal characteristic which is needed to give the embryo a claim to consideration is sentience, or the capacity to feel pain or pleasure. Until the embryo reaches that point, there is nothing we can do to the embryo which causes harm to *it*. We can, of course, damage it in such a way as to cause harm to the person it will become, if it lives, but if it never becomes a person, the embryo has not been harmed, because its total lack of awareness means that it can have no interest in becoming a person.

Once an embryo may be capable of feeling pain, there is a clear case for very strict controls over the experimentation which can be done with it. At this point the embryo ranks, morally, with other creatures who are conscious but not self-conscious. Many nonhuman animals come into this category, and in my view they have often been unjustifiably made to suffer in scientific research. We should have stringent controls over research to ensure that this cannot happen to embryos, just as we should have stringent controls to ensure that it cannot happen to animals.

Practical Implications of the Moral Status of Embryos

The conclusion to draw from this is that as long as the parents give their consent, there is no ethical objection to discarding a very early embryo. If the early embryo can be used for significant research, so much the better. What is crucial is that the embryo not be kept beyond the point at which it has formed a brain and a nervous system, and might be capable of suffering. Two government committees—the Warnock Committee in Britain (8) and the Waller Committee in Victoria, Australia (9)—have recently recommended that research on embryos should be allowed, but only up to 14 days after fertilization. This is the period at which the so-called "primitive streak," the first indication of the development of a nervous system, begins to form, and up to this stage there is certainly no possibility of the embryo feeling anything at all. In fact, the 14-day limit is unnecessarily conservative. A limit of, say, 28 days would still be very much on the safe side of the best estimates of when the embryo may be able to feel pain; but such a limit would, in contrast to the 14-day limit, allow research on embryos at the stage at which some of the more specialized cells have begun to form. As we saw earlier, this research would, according to Robert Edwards, have the potential to cure such terrible diseases as sickle cell anemia and leukemia (2).

As for freezing the embryo with a view to later implantation, the question here is essentially one of risk. If freezing carries no special risk of abnormality, there seems to be nothing objectionable about it. With embryo freezing, this appears to be the case. The ethical objections some people have to freezing embryos has led to the suggestion that it would be better to freeze eggs (8); for this and other reasons there has been a considerable research effort directed at freezing eggs. Human eggs are more difficult to freeze than human embryos, and until recently it had not proved possible to freeze them in a manner which allowed fertilization after thawing. In December 1985, however, an IVF team at Flinders University, in Adelaide, South Australia, announced that it had succeeded in obtaining a pregnancy from an egg which had been frozen and thawed before being fertilized (10). The technique used involved stripping away a protective outer layer from the egg, so that it would take up a chemical which would protect it during the freezing process. This technique does overcome the ethical problems some find in freezing embryos, but it does so at the cost of introducing a new potential cause of risk to the offspring, the risk that the chemicals absorbed by the egg may have some harmful effect (11). Whether or not this risk proves to be a real one, from the point of view of ethics, one may doubt whether the risk is worth running, if the primary reason for running it is to avoid objections, which we have now seen to be ill-founded, to the freezing of embryos.

Going beyond the simple case does bring us into a more ethically controversial area, but there is no overall case against applying IVF outside the restricted ambit of the simple case. The essential point is to consider each additional step carefully before it is taken. Some steps will prove unwise, but others will be beneficial and not open to any well-grounded objections.

The Future of the Reproduction Revolution

What lies ahead? IVF has opened the door to a wide range of further possibilities. In the near future we shall have to consider which of these possibilities to pursue, and which to reject. Here are some of the possibilities:

1. A surrogate could bear a child for another couple; the child would be the genetic child of the other couple, and would be returned to the genetic parents after birth. The genetic parents might be unable to conceive in the normal way, or they might simply find the surrogate arrangement more convenient. The surrogate might be paid for her services, or—in the case of otherwise infertile couples—she may have more altruistic motives.

2. Embryos may be used in order to provide "spare parts" for people who through accident or illness need some kind of transplant. It has been suggested that embryonic tissue could restore nerve function to paraplegics. Embryos might be grown to the point at which the organs begin to form, and then the organs could be separated and grown in culture until they were large enough to be used.

3. Several embryos could be produced, and some of their genetic characteristics identified; the one considered most desirable could then be implanted, and the remainder discarded; alternatively it will eventually be possible to modify the genetic properties of an embryo so as to eliminate defects and to build in desirable genetic qualities.

There are other possibilities too, but it is enough if we confine ourselves to these. Let us start with surrogate motherhood. Surrogate motherhood using artificial insemination is already a reality. In the United States, it is being practiced commercially, though still on a small scale. In Britain, in the aftermath of the much publicized Baby Cotton case, Parliament moved swiftly to prohibit commercial agencies getting involved in surrogacy, but the new law did not affect the parties to the arrangement themselves. Thus people remained free to arrange their own surrogacies, if they wished, and even to pay for a surrogate, as long as no agency was involved. Whatever we think of this kind of surrogacy (that is, surrogacy not using IVF), it is not going to be possible to stop it, since it does not require the services of a medical practitioner. The best we can do is to regulate it and to try to eliminate some of the obvious problems: women who are psychologically unprepared for surrogacy and wish to keep the baby; women who are prepared to threaten to abort the baby in order to extract more money from the infertile couple; and couples who refuse to accept the baby if it is born with a defect.

Surrogacy with IVF is not so different, except that it may be a little easier, psychologically, for the surrogate to part with a baby who is not her genetic child. On the other hand, the number of couples who would be interested in using a surrogate will no doubt increase if the child can be the genetic child of both parents. It would, of course, be easier to prohibit surrogacy using IVF, since this does require sophisticated medical services; but there are at least some cases in which surrogacy may benefit all parties and harm none, for instance cases in which a friend or relative offers to help an infertile couple. Where there is no commercial motivation, problems seem likely to be fewer, and adequate counseling should be able to overcome most of the difficulties.

A commercial system of surrogacy raises much greater problems. It threatens to divide our society into the poor who bear children and the rich who have others do it for them. This may bring economic benefits to the poor, but at considerable psychological cost. Perhaps some regulated system of commercial surrogacy may eventually be judged acceptable, but for the present it would seem best to restrict surrogacy to cases in which the motivation is altruistic and any payment is limited to the reimbursement of genuine expenses incurred as a result of the pregnancy.

The proposal that embryos be used for "spare parts" has already caused howls of protest from those who regard embryos as having the same rights as normal human beings. We have seen, however, that this view cannot be defended by rational argument. As long as there are adequate safeguards to ensure that the embryo is at all times incapable of suffering in any way, it is difficult to find sound ethical reason against this proposal—and it is obvious that the possible benefits are considerable.

Of all the possible applications of IVF, however, it is genetic selection and genetic engineering which raise the most far-reaching questions. Should we tinker with the human genetic pool? If so, in what way? Here I will limit myself to pointing out that we already tinker with the genetic pool when we offer genetic counseling, amniocentesis, and abortion to those who are at special risk of producing genetically defective offspring. And this is nothing new, at least insofar as its impact on the genetic pool is concerned: other societies have practiced infanticide to the same end, and of course in the past, even if one tried to rear the defective child, in most cases nature used its own brutal methods to ensure that the genes were eliminated from the gene pool.

So genetic engineering differs only in its techniques from what is now going on, and has gone on for a long time. But this difference is a significant one, because the new techniques are so much more powerful, and because they would, in principle, allow us to select for desirable traits as well as to select against undesirable ones. Many fear that these techniques will place too much power in the hands of governments, who will not be able to resist the temptation of designing future generations to be docile and to vote for the governing party at every election.

The fear that genetic engineering will produce the ultimate in entrenched dictatorship is exaggerated. Most political leaders want quick results, and it would take at least 18 years for genetic engineering to have any effect at the polls. If we have succeeded in keeping our freedom in the age of television and state education, we should be able to cling to it in the age of genetic engineering as well.

But should we allow positive modifications, as distinct from the elimination of defects, at all? In time we might come to accept the desirability of positive modifications. One reason for accepting this is that, looking around us, there is reason to think that natural selection has left ample room for improvement. Another reason is that the distinction between eliminating a defect and making a positive modification is a difficult one to draw. If we learn how to eliminate a wide range of defects which predispose us to common diseases, we will have created an abnormally healthy person. If we learn how to affect intelligence, should we stop short at eliminating mental ability below the above-average range? If we eliminate abnormally depressive personalities, would it be wrong to try to produce people who tend to be a little more cheerful than most of us are now? If we eliminate tendencies toward criminal violence, might we not build just a little more kindness into the human constitution? If the risks of such an enterprise are great, so too are the potential rewards for us all.

References

1. Singer P, Wells D. Making babies. New York: Scribner's, 1985.
2. Edwards RG. Paper presented at the Fourth World Congress on IVF. Melbourne, Australia, Nov 22, 1985.
3. Abstract. Proceedings of the Fifth Scientific Meeting of the Fertility Society of Australia, Adelaide, Dec. 2–6, 1986.

4. Rowland R. Reproductive technologies: the final solution to the woman question? In: Arditti R, Klein RD, Minden S, eds, Test-tube women: what future for motherhood? London: Pandora, 1984.

5. Firestone S. The dialectic of sex. New York: Bantam, 1971.

6. Breeze N. Who is going to rock the petri dish? In: Arditti R, Klein RD, Minden S, eds, Test-tube women: what future for motherhood? London: Pandora, 1984.

7. Glover J. Causing death and saving lives. Harmondsworth, England: Penguin, 1977.

8. Warnock M (Chairperson). Report of the Committee of Inquiry into Human Fertilisation and Embryology. London: Her Majesty's Stationery Office, 1984, p 66.

9. Waller L (Chairman). Victorian Government Committee to Consider the Social, Ethical and Legal Issues Arising from In Vitro Fertilization. Report on the disposition of embryos produced by in vitro fertilization. Melbourne: Victorian Government Printer, 1984, p 47.

10. The Australian, Dec 19, 1985.

11. Trounson A. Paper presented at the Fourth World Congress on IVF, Melbourne, Australia, Nov 22, 1985.

3

Ethical Issues in Genetic Screening, Prenatal Diagnosis, and Counseling

JOHN C. FLETCHER

In contemporary societies, genetic assessments occur in the context of genetic screening, prenatal diagnosis, and genetic counseling. This chapter will discuss some ethical issues in these areas. The discussion will 1) identify the major moral or value-laden problems parents, practitioners, and policymakers have faced and will face in the near future, 2) describe varying ethical positions taken on the problems, and 3) (as I was invited to) argue for my own positions on the issues.

Familiar ethical issues will be distinguished from the unfamiliar. The distinction between familiar and unfamiliar is descriptive and historical, rather than normative. When a body of experience and literature collects around an issue which arises frequently in practice, and when an approach to the *ethical* aspects of the issue is shaped and gradually selected, the issue can be characterized as familiar, even though it is still difficult and controversial. Unfamiliar ethical issues are those new to the field, prior to serious study, debate, or testing of approaches.

Some authors categorize prenatal diagnosis as genetic screening because the goal is to obtain information about the genotype of the fetus (1, 2). In my view, ethical reasons prompt a sharper distinction between genetic screening and prenatal diagnosis, because the pregnant woman's safety and welfare and the father's interests in her safety and the fetus are morally relevant differences that distinguish prenatal diagnosis from genetic screening involving separate persons like newborns, carriers, family members, and other nonpregnant populations.

Ethical considerations in present and prospective treatment of genetic disorders will be discussed briefly in the section on prenatal diagnosis. More complete discussions of the state of the art and ethics of treatment of genetic disorders can be found elsewhere (3, 4).

This chapter reflects the views of the author and does not represent official policies or positions of the National Institutes of Health.

Correspondence and reprint requests should be directed to Dr. Fletcher, Building 10, Room 2C-202, NIH, Bethesda, MD 20892.

Medical geneticists, interdisciplinary groups, official ethics commissions, and authorities in ethics have created a very large body of literature on ethics and human genetics. Statements of policy and ethical guidance have gradually evolved for practitioners (5–10). Each section in this chapter concludes with a condensed statement of ethical guidance for the most frequent and familiar ethical problems faced by practitioners, parents, and policymakers. Allowing for some cultural differences, medical geneticists are likely to concur with these statements, although this hypothesis needs to be tested (11).

Beyond familiar ethical problems lie many difficult and novel issues precipitated by technical progress in DNA technology used to map the human genome (12). Concurrently, interest is growing in genetic research in the human zygote and developing embryo (13, 14). A looming agenda of unfamiliar ethical problems looms which needs wider debate in a societally approved forum. New moral pathways must be found and boundaries drawn to guide the use of such techniques for genetic diagnosis and eventual treatment of genetic disorders. The final section summarizes these newer issues and the questions for debate.

Genetic Screening

The general objective of genetic screening is to test an asymptomatic population to discover persons with a particular genotype. Historically, genetic screening has extended its scope as follows:
1.   newborn screening for medical interventions
2.   carrier screening for reproductive choices
3.   screening for susceptibility to common diseases
4.   screening in the workplace
5.   research

Screening can precede the delivery of medical care, especially to affected homozygotes, for the harmful consequences of genetic disorders. Screening of newborns to detect phenylketonuria (PKU) and prevent significant mental retardation by a low phenylalanine diet began in the early 1960s. PKU has a low incidence (1 in 11,500), but a devastating result if untreated. The ease of detection, despite the complexities of the disease itself, has led to virtually universal screening in developed countries. Today, many newborns are also tested for hypothyroidism (1 in 4,000), which can be successfully treated by thyroid hormone replacement. Less frequent screening occurs for galactosemia, maple syrup urine disease, homocystinuria, and sickle cell disease.

Carriers can obviously benefit from knowledge of their health histories, especially in their reproductive choices and prior to marriage. Carrier screening can be informative to couples about hitherto unknown risks they bring to reproduction and reduce harm in their families. Large-scale screening programs have been carried out in Ashkenazic Jewish communities (1 in 30 at risk) to detect carriers of Tay-Sachs disease, in black communities (1 in 12 at risk) to detect carriers of sickle cell disease, and in many Mediterranean communities to detect carriers of thalassemia. Screening for heterozygotes for cystic fibrosis, the most common lethal genetic disease in the United States, remains an elusive goal. About 1 in 20 whites and 1 in 60 blacks in the United States carries the cystic fibrosis gene.

Familiar Ethical Problems in Genetic Screening

Three ethical problems occurred in the early stage of large-scale carrier screening and, to a lesser extent, in newborn screening: unjustifiably harmful or coercive practices, problems of confidentiality, and stigmatization of persons at higher genetic risk. Steps were taken subsequently to construct clearer guidelines to protect participants and to define ethically justifiable goals. However, some moral criticisms of genetic screening programs continue to be made for one or more of these reasons.

Harmful or Coercive Practices

A National Academy of Sciences Committee for the Study of Errors of Inborn Metabolism concluded that "hindsight reveals that screening programs for phenylketonuria were instituted before the validity and effectiveness of all aspects of treatment, including appropriate dietary treatment, were thoroughly tested" (6: p. 2). Direct harm was done to some children with phenylalanine depletion who were screened and treated by dietary regulation when mandatory screening practices were initiated in the early to mid-1960s. Some remote or indirect harm could have been done to children with a form of hyperphenylalinemia who were also screened and treated. The latter children were not, in fact, destined to become retarded.

The early history of screening for sickle cell trait also reveals premature, harmful, and coercive practices. Beginning in 1970, many state legislators and community leaders rushed to frame laws mandating screening for black children and at least one state required adults to be tested prior to issuance of a marriage license (15). Part of the motivation to screen was based on confusion about the difference between the sickle trait and the disease itself. Indeed, medical literature itself saw such confusion in an editorial that referred to screening "22 million

Afro-Americans" for a "dread disease" (16). A period of actual chaos ensued in many urban communities in which mandatory screening began without informed consent. Positive results obtained from carrier tests were misinterpreted as evidence of disease by parents who had not had proper counseling. In this period, the deaths of four black recruits in training was linked to the sickle cell trait (17). Congress debated barring black youths with sickle cell carrier trait from military service. Some black sickle cell carriers were unjustly barred from sports, denied employment, and even discharged from jobs (18). By the time efforts were made to define goals for screening and to clear the air of confusion, damage had been done to the cause of screening for sickle cell trait (19).

In 1972 the passage of the National Sickle Cell Anemia Control Act authorized funds only to state programs premised on voluntary participation. Each law requiring genetic screening was rescinded or ignored. Between 1972 and 1983 an interdisciplinary task force of the Hastings Center, a committee of the National Academy of Sciences, and a President's Commission stressed the voluntariness of genetic screening and the priority of the personal wishes, choices, and actions of the persons to be screened (5–7). None of these working groups found any justification for compulsory genetic screening except to prevent serious harm to the newborn, and they found no compelling arguments for screening based on a "healthy gene pool" or cost-benefit considerations.

Some moral critics of genetic screening are not persuaded by arguments for voluntarism and parental use of information as the main goal of screening. Since screening involves ethnic identification of groups already vulnerable for religious and racial prejudice, the practice invites criticism. Even after glowing reports of community cooperation, Goodman and Goodman still found Tay-Sachs screening among Jews to have an "invidious effect" because it limited the freedom of a target population and targeted one group to the exclusion of others (20). In spite of their recognition of the benefits of screening, a Roman Catholic study of genetic screening programs saw dangers of universally mandated screening, the dominance of the state over reproductive decisions, and economic and social intolerance of affected persons and those who refused to participate in screening (21).

Confidentiality Problems

The three groups to examine the ethics of screening held that it should be defined primarily as a medical procedure in the context of the physician-patient relationship, even though carrier screening often occurs in community settings. Protection of patient confidentiality is a major feature of medical ethics. However, in the early days of carrier screening for sickle cell trait, there were many examples of unrelated third parties, like employers and insurers, being given results of screening under the misunderstanding that the participant was at higher risk for disease. The practice was strengthened to withhold results of screening from interested third parties contingent upon the explicit consent of the patient.

This clear restriction does not always apply, however, in some dilemmas about disclosure that arise in screening. Medical geneticists are sometimes faced with cases in which patients refuse to allow information or test results to be shared with relatives who may themselves be at risk. Also, screening may reveal nonpaternity. In this event, the welfare of the mother and the unity of the family and the marriage are of serious concern. These dilemmas occur in the context of both screening and prenatal diagnosis, but the approaches charted by medical geneticists will be described at the end of this section.

Stigmatization

Stigmatization is a complex social interaction that results in labeling, social distance, and lowered feelings of self-esteem (22). Kenen and Schmidt reviewed the risk of stigmatization of carrier status resulting from the psychological, social, and economic consequences of screening programs. They defined stigmatization as "feelings of inadequacy or strangeness that are themselves damaging to health" (23: p. 1117). Goodman and Goodman defined stigmatization as the association of "a certain group or an individual . . . with negative social or psychological characteristics" (20: p. 24) that weakens self-image, results in difficulty of finding marriage partners, and provides a self-fulfilling prophecy for those who want scientific grounds to hold ancient prejudices against a group like Jews. Massarik and Kayback found latitude in the concept of stigma being applied to screening that ranged from "deeply incisive and damaging imprints of a physiologic or psychologic nature . . . to a transient state of discomfort and concern" (24).

The consequences of stigmatization were indeed found in a followup of a 1972 sickle cell screening program in a small Greek village where carrier frequency was 23 percent and newborn disease occurred in 1 of 100 births (25). Because the village population was so attuned to genetic risks, some disruption of social existence followed screening. Engagements to marry were broken and stigma was manifested by women who lied to prospective marriage partners about genetic status. Also, four carrier-carrier marriages took place after screening. These discouraging results made the program seem futile.

Clow and Scriver found that 10 percent of 45 detected carriers in a population of Canadian high school students screened for Tay-Sachs trait described a "diminished self-image," while about the same number of noncarriers stated an "improvement" in self-image (26). About 88 percent of heterozygotes said that their self-image was unchanged but that their parents were "worried" about the results. Two other evaluations of the feelings of carriers following screening for Tay-Sachs and thalassemia trait clearly showed the variable psychological impact of the new knowledge and created a good reason to be concerned about the mental health of a small number of persons who were most disturbed (27, 28).

No comprehensive study of social stigmatization and genetic screening in a developed country has been fully carried out. However, a follow-up study eight years after screening a high school population for Tay-Sachs carrier trait showed that anxiety diminished with time and that most discussed the knowledge with significant others and sought genetic counseling if their partner was also a heterozygote (29). In my view, the data show a small but clear risk of stigmatization which obligates geneticists to attempt to identify those at greatest risk and take precautions to modify or prevent the most harmful results.

Will stigmatization increase with the extension of the scope of genetic screening? As more screening occurs among heterozygotes, more knowledge will spread about the ubiquity of genetic risks. No ethnic group can take pride in its lack of genetic problems. If many in different ethnic groups know their risks, less opportunity exists to promote invidious comparisons or punitive attitudes. As genetic services are made available to more persons, the perception of being trapped in a punishing biological prison will be reduced and carriers will be less apt to hold negative views of themselves for long periods. This view is also supported by the lack of evidence of social ostracism or punishment of those who, found to be at higher genetic risk, choose not to use screening or prenatal diagnosis. A society in which ostracism of nonusers of genetic services finds little fertile soil is unlikely to abet stigmatization if genetic screening expands to new groups of carriers.

Genetic Susceptibility to Disease

In 1972, to avert the misuse of genetic knowledge derived from carrier screening, a guideline of the Genetics Research Group of the Hastings Center asserted: "It is unjustifiable to promulgate standards for normalcy based on genetic constitution" (5). In 1984 a coauthor of these guidelines, Lappe, wrote that this injunction needs "to be tempered with a new reality," because with new techniques for DNA analysis, "it is now possible to define the 'normal' (that is, most prevalent) genotype with great precision, and to use direct measurements of genes to define the likelihood of pending disease" (30). Curiously, Lappe misquoted the Hastings guideline. In his words it reads: "genetic data should not be used as criteria for normalcy." The aim of the Hastings statement in 1972 was to prevent the labeling of a carrier as "abnormal." Further, it aimed to criticize hasty state lawmakers whose promulgations implied that carriers were sick or deviant. An example was Massachusetts, Chapter 491 of Acts and Resolves (July 1, 1971), "requiring the testing of blood for sickle trait or anemia as a prerequisite to school attendance."

A redraft of the Hastings guideline today might better read: "It is unjustifiable to promulgate standards of *societal* normalcy based on genetic constitution." The guideline probably helped to prevent stigmatization, unfair labeling, and coercion of carriers of recessive genes. But if Lappe believes today that the Hastings statement meant that genetic data should not be used as criteria to assess the *health status* of individuals, families, and populations, he is projecting a contemporary issue into the past. However, genetic data are increasingly vital for the assessment of health status, as Lappe's current discussion shows.

Genetic data derived by the use of probes that locate genetic markers on restriction fragment-length polymorphisms will greatly increase the scope of genetic screening of individuals whose genotypes render them susceptible to disease. Research in DNA-assisted techniques is steadily increasing to enable presymptomatic diagnosis of homozygotes with Huntington's disease, muscular dystrophy, cystic fibrosis, and familial hypercholesterolemia, to mention only some major disorders (31–34). Genetic information is newly available about many cancers that may clearly lend itself to earlier diagnosis and genetic assessment in families at higher risk for cancer (35). These conditions represent a spectrum of disorders from lethal and untreatable to treatable by surgery or diet. Whether research on genetic susceptibility to cancer will also reveal genetic approaches to cancer treatment is unclear. At the outer edges of the spectrum are examples of known health risks to heterozygotes in hypercholesterolemia, Fanconi's anemia, X-linked mental retardation, and sickle cell disease (36).

These advances create at least two unfamiliar ethical problems. First, family members and physicians will face the questions of whether, when, and how persons should learn that they have a lethal and untreatable genetic disorder. The issues involved in disclosure will be especially difficult in children and unemancipated minors. Families at risk for

Huntington's disease will probably be the first to face these questions (37).

The second problem faces society and policymakers: how will an early detected "victim," especially one with an untreatable disorder, be protected from genetic discrimination? Without some controls on disclosure to unrelated third parties, knowledge of impending serious disease in spheres of education, employment, and insurance would lead to isolation, loss of opportunities, and excessively high insurance premiums for the vulnerable individual. Will the insured at lower genetic risks be willing to absorb the lifetime costs of medical care for those at the highest levels of susceptibility? Are not some employers, such as airlines and other industries involved with public safety, entitled to know about the health status of employees who may be risks to that safety, even though a genetic disease is the primary source of that threat? These are serious problems for which society is not prepared.

Lappe believes that the protection of human subjects' confidentiality and autonomy that has evolved in the ethics of research will serve in the present interim between research to develop screening methods and the application of that research in medical practice (30). New work in mapping the human genome by DNA techniques shrinks the length of the interim with each passing month. No effective controls exist to protect those who want to know their medical destiny and to live as responsibly as possible with that knowledge. How this potentially damaging information should be managed, by whom, and for what purposes needs to be debated and clarified in a wider social forum as soon as possible.

Genetic Screening in the Workplace

Genetic monitoring in the workplace should be distinguished from genetic screening of workers (38). The former involves the periodic testing of employees for evidence of damage to their DNA or chromosomes from toxic agents or hazards. The latter entails screening workers for genetic traits believed to involve higher susceptibility to diseases complicated by workplace hazards. Probably more genetic screening of workers took place in the 1960s and 1970s than occurs today. The first reports that glucose-6-phosphate dehydrogenase (G-6-PD) deficiency was possibly involved in anemias of workers with chemicals were in the early 1960s (39, 40). In 1963 Stokinger and Mountain listed 37 known chemicals that caused hemolysis to which workers with G-6-PD deficiency may have been susceptible (41). Consequently, by 1967 at least 15 industries screened for G-6-PD (42). Other examples of risks of genetic susceptibility can be studied in specific workplaces: does the cystic fibrosis carrier suffer excessively from gastric-duodenal ulceration and bronchial infections (43)? Are alpha 1 antitrypsin deficiency carriers at a higher risk for pulmonary disease (44)? Do some "normal genes" whose products can be recognized, interacting with specific environmental conditions, influence susceptibility to common diseases (45)? Such health risks might be higher in some workplaces.

Expert medical opinion is that all genetic screening tests applied to workers are *research* procedures and should not be done routinely (46). Genetic screening in the workplace is an applied science in an early stage of evolution. In occupational diseases, genetic factors are probably one of a number of predisposing factors including age, overall health status, and nutrition. However, despite the wide degree of genetic variation involved in such problems, an impressive body of evidence exists that genotype can be correlated with some occupational diseases (47). At present political and legal problems, as well as ethical questions that cannot be resolved until a more solid scientific foundation for worker screening exists, have blunted an energetic approach to the many scientific and epidemiological problems that need attention.

In 1980 it was reported that the Du Pont Company was screening black workers for sickle cell trait (48). Congressional hearings about screening workers followed in 1981 and led to a study of the prevalence of genetic screening of workers by the Office of Technology Assessment (38: pp. 33–40). Questionnaires were sent to the chief executive officers of the 500 largest industrial companies, and their counterparts in the 50 largest private utility companies and 11 major unions representing the largest numbers of workers in these companies. Responses (366) from corporations, unions, and utilities showed 5 currently using genetic screening, 12 that had used it in the past, and 54 stating that screening would be considered in the future if tests were proved to be reliable. Screening for sickle cell trait had been done by 10 organizations, but the purpose of such screening was very unclear. Since this period, corporations have been very quiet about screening practices and have probably discouraged its use.

Murray gave the most thorough, and in most respects, balanced ethical analysis of prospective genetic screening in the workplace (49, 50). He saw four purposes of worker screening: diagnosis, research, information, and exclusion. Each purpose was defined in an ascending scale of ethical constraints, diagnosis of disease requiring the least and any policy to exclude workers at higher risk from specific jobs needing maximum constraint. Murray pointed to three possibly negative consequences of diagnosis: 1) blaming the person and exonerating workplace

conditions, 2) labeling the sick person, and 3) creating difficulty in finding another job.

Murray noted the need for epidemiological research on the links
between populations of workers, workplace exposures, and illness. If
these links are established, new studies of the effectiveness of screening
to prevent or reduce illness should follow. During the interim of research, vital questions arise as to how the best interests of worker-
subjects can be protected, and how research data can be protected until
associations between genes, working conditions, and illness are proved
or disproved. These questions must be settled before on-the-job screening or screening of prospective workers can take place routinely.

Any exclusionary policy, in Murray's view, needs to be based on an
"absolute" requirement of a proven linkage between genotype, exposure, and disease. He adds several "conditional" requirements: very
large risks, few false positives or negatives which need to be reversible,
small numbers of people involved, very few jobs involved, severe and
irreversible disease, and screening should not single out already vulnerable groups.

Two flaws appear in Murray's reasoning. In establishing scientifically valid proof of links between human genes and workplace hazards,
a criterion of "absolute" scientific certainty is impossible to attain. A
very high standard of probability is within the realm of the possible. An
impossible scientific standard could be morally self-defeating and prevent protection of workers from harm. Also, Murray's insistence that
"few jobs" must be involved seems less important ethically than preventing harm to workers, especially when the risks of harm are known
to be "very large." Subordinating great damage to health to holding a
job, even when many jobs are involved, is not ethically sound. To provide security to workers being screened, industries need to assure that
three conditions precede a policy of exclusion from jobs based upon
genetic susceptibility: 1) workers screened on the job who test positive
will not lose employment but will be offered or retrained for other opportunities, 2) applicants for jobs with hazards heightened by genetic
susceptibility will be informed and consent to a requirement for screening prior to employment, and 3) an aggressive program to reduce risks
in the workplace already exists.

Ethical Guidelines for Genetic Screening

On the basis of preexisting statements (5–7, 11), practitioners and
policymakers would likely agree with the following guidelines for
genetic screening:

1.   Any mandatory approach to genetic screening, except for new-born screening for treatable disorders, is ethically objectionable and counterproductive. An individual's choice not to be screened for genetic reasons should be respected and no pressure exerted.

2.   Large-scale screening programs for heterozygote conditions should not be implemented until their value has first been demonstrated in well-conducted pilot studies.

3.   School-age and preschool children should not be routinely screened for carrier status in organized programs. Screening at preadolescence or in adolescence confers more benefit for reproductive choices and planning.

4.   Information from genetic testing should be given to third parties only with the explicit consent of the person screened.

5.   The strongest, most effective state-of-the-art methods should be used to protect genetic-related information in data banks of private and government agencies.

6.   When patients refuse to allow test results to be shared with relatives who may themselves be at risk, a duty of confidentiality exists, but it may be overridden in some circumstances by the need to prevent harm to others. These conditions are relevant before breaching confidentiality: a) reasonable efforts to persuade the patient to voluntary consent of disclosure have failed, b) a high probability exists both that harm will occur if information is withheld and that the disclosed information will actually be used to avert harm, c) the harm that others would suffer would be serious, and d) precautions are taken to ensure that only the genetic information needed for diagnosis and treatment of the disease in question is disclosed.

7.   In findings that strongly suggest that the putative father is not the biological father of the child, and when the facts of the case must unavoidably be disclosed because of genetic risks, physicians should meet first with the mother to advise her of the finding. They should recommend special care to help her with her choice about disclosure and the process of any future genetic counseling. The choices about disclosure are the woman's and should be safeguarded.

8.   When reliable tests for presymptomatic detections of serious genetic disorders, such as Huntington's disease, become firmly established, they should be made available to families and individuals at risk, provided proper support and counseling precede and accompany their use. Medical geneticists ought to help to design an optimal approach to disclosure and be prepared to work closely with other physicians and mental health specialists familiar with the needs and problems in these families. In cases where children or unemancipated minors are in-

volved, the parents' desires should prevail about disclosure, after sufficient counseling has been provided about the potential consequences
and to test the family's ability to cope.

9.   Future genetic screening to identify persons more susceptible to
common diseases and workplace harms should be accompanied by measures to protect the individual from stigmatization, misuse of information by third parties, and discharge from employment because of genetic
risks alone. Medical geneticists should participate in designing rules for
the handling of data concerning disease susceptibility.

Ethical Issues in Prenatal Diagnosis

Four familiar ethical problems in prenatal diagnosis will be discussed:
abortion choices, controversial indications, problems in disclosure of
diagnostic results, and problems of access and distribution of services. A
historical survey of these issues is available elsewhere in the context of
reviews of the state-of-the-art of prenatal diagnosis, its utilization and
consequences (51).

First trimester diagnosis by chorionic villus sampling (CVS) is the
most important technical advance in prenatal diagnosis since midtrimester amniocentesis was introduced in the United States as applied research in 1967. The safety and accuracy of CVS compared to amniocentesis is being studied in trials in several nations (52). CVS should be
regarded as applied research until controlled clinical trials provide reliable evidence of its value.

Can genetic assessment be pushed even farther back to the preimplantation human embryo? Despite serious technical problems and potential dangers to the embryo, interest is growing in this question (13, 14,
53). Genetic assessment would reach its ultimate horizon if human gametes from parents or donors could be selected to avoid harmful genes,
although a method of diagnosis that would not also harm or kill the sex
cells is difficult to imagine. One great ethical advantage of gametic selection would be the avoidance of genetic abortions. Given present social
and economic inequalities, however, one great disadvantage could well
be unfair distribution of such services, with large consequences for dif-
ferentials for health in different social classes. Unfamiliar and difficult
ethical issues arise about the potential uses and timing of prenatal diagnosis and its links to techniques of *in vitro* fertilization (IVF) and embryo
transfer (ET), which need study and debate.

Abortion Choices

Positive findings occur in approximately 4.4 percent of total amniocentesis procedures performed (54). Faced with a finding of disease, parents

have these choices: to abort, to try fetal therapy in rare instances, to wait until delivery and treat the infant if possible, or to arrange for adoption or foster parent procedures after delivery. Current practice is to allow diversity and parental choices to prevail.

Although most parents who use prenatal diagnosis choose to abort if results are positive, such choices present difficult ethical dilemmas. Dilemmas are posed by 1) views of the higher moral status of the fetus at midtrimester, 2) the wide spectrum of severity in some diagnosable genetic disorders, 3) the ability to treat some disorders, and 4) cases of twins where one is diagnosed as affected.

The Moral Status of the Midtrimester Fetus

Abortion at midtrimester is morally problematic because the fetus at midtrimester is thought by many to have a significantly higher moral status than the fetus in the first trimester. Some older and newer modes of ethical thought about abortion embody a developmental view of the moral status of the fetus. Not until the nineteenth century did the view appear that the interests of the newly fertilized embryo are morally equal to those of each living human being (55, 56). Pope Pius IX, impressed with new knowledge about human embryogenesis, ruled that fertilization was the moment of full humanhood. An older moral tradition based on views of "animation" or "ensoulment" of the fetus has more in common with a developmental view than a categorical view of embryonic and fetal equality, although views that stress fetal equality have clearly gained ground in recent years.

Some physicians and ethicists claim that prenatal diagnosis is associated with an intrinsic ethical flaw, in that genetic assessment sets apart certain fetuses as deserving of abortion, thus treating them unequally and unjustly. Kass argued that to single out defective fetuses for abortion on the basis of arbitrary and changeable social and personal reasons violated the belief in the moral equality of all human beings (57). Lejeune began from a view of the biological unity of mankind to object to the condemnation of specific damaged fetuses. In his view, one would be intrinsically wrong to interrupt biological continuity for abortion of any fetus, regardless of the consequences (58). Ramsey also affirmed the right of the diseased fetus to equal protection and patienthood, and like Kass, argued that one could not logically arrive at a moral justification for genetic abortion that could not also be used to justify infanticide and neglect of the handicapped (59).

Key differences between ethical perspectives on abortion after prenatal diagnosis turn on the question of the moral status of the fetus. Other authorities in ethics and medicine who take a developmental view draw boundaries that permit abortion for serious and untreatable disorders (60–63). A developmental view refers to, but is not determined by, biological milestones in embryonic and fetal development. Developmental physiology is a partner for moral reasoning about abortion choices, but the ethical principles that guide choice encourage respect for the life and potential personhood of the fetus at each point in the development of an increasingly recognizable human being. The more the fetus grows to possess some recognizable human features and crucial biological capacities, the more the moral status of the fetus approximates that of living persons. These views encourage reasoning that balances fetal interests with those of mother, parents, and family. Indifference toward fetal life at any stage of development is not ethically acceptable.

Abortion after amniocentesis is performed most frequently between 18 and 21 weeks of gestation. At this point the human fetus has a clearly recognizable human form easily seen by parents and physicians via ultrasonography. The fetus has also passed some important biological milestones in the development of a central nervous system and other organs and is close to the stage at which very premature infants might be kept alive. Each characteristic encourages acceptance of a higher moral status of the developing fetus, but still would not, in current public policy, be sufficient grounds to overrule the choice of parents to abort after positive findings.

Parents suffer emotionally before and after genetic abortion. Four of five studies document acute emotional trauma and depression in many couples and especially in the woman (64–68). Do parents suffer morally as well? That is, when they choose abortion do they impose moral guilt upon themselves from having violated values and principles affirming a high moral status of the fetus? The moral experience of parents, their views of the moral status of the fetus, and their reasoning about their abortion choices have not been studied as well as the emotional sequelae to genetic abortions have. Findings on long-term effects in four of five studies tend to agree with the conclusion of a thorough follow-up of 20 patients: "The decision to terminate a second trimester pregnancy because of a malformed fetus is an event with long term negative side-effects for the patient and the family" (66). Research is needed that compares the emotional and moral aspects of second and first trimester abortion for genetic indications. Presumably, the degree of emotional and moral suffering would be less following the CVS experience.

Wide Spectrum of Severity

If the degree of severity of a fetal disorder could be known in each case with certainty, a morally relevant line could be drawn to separate the most severe cases where abortion is morally justified and the least severe in which the grounds for abortion are less weighty. Wide degrees of severity are present in genetic disorders. Precise information cannot, however, be given the parents about how severely the fetus will be affected. Abortion choices must now be made informed only by the statistical range of severity. Since knowledge of serious and untreatable harm to the fetus is the strongest ethical reason that justifies genetic abortion, when uncertainty prevails about severity the abortion choice would be very difficult.

On one side of severity, de la Chappelle wrote of the formidable challenge of a chromosomal diagnosis of 47 XYY to counselee and counselor alike (69). Different facts about this disorder can be taken in different ways. One may emphasize that the child will appear normal until the age of 12. One can also stress the real risk of mild mental retardation, emotional difficulty, and antisocial behavior in later life. Both are true, but is this chromosomal abnormality sufficiently severe to warrant abortion? In such cases, the prevailing rule is to respect the views of the parents, after a thorough explanation has been given of the potential and the problems that such children present.

At the other end of the spectrum, anencephaly is a diagnosable disorder incompatible with life. Ethicists like Haering and Ramsey usually take positions strongly defending the sanctity of life in abortion and newborn care. Nevertheless, they except anencephaly because of the virtually total forebrain deficit (70, 71). Chervenak and others discussed the moral justification of abortion in the third trimester (72). They found anencephaly the only condition that clearly met their two necessary criteria: 1) a disorder that is a) incompatible with postnatal survival for more than a few weeks, or b) marked by the total or virtual absence of cognitive function; and 2) reliable diagnostic procedures for determining that the condition of the fetus meets either of these two criteria.

Powars described the spectrum of severity in sickle cell disease (73). Ten percent of those born with the disease will die in the first decade of life. Peak morbidity is between the second and third years. However, some patients have only slight infections and minor pain controllable by aspirin. Research in prenatal diagnosis of sickle cell disease is being focused on measurement of the severity of the disease, in the hope of helping parents make abortion choices that embody more accurate estimates of severity (74).

Status of Treatment of Genetic Disorders

Treatability of genetic disorders before or after birth is the source of a second moral line to help distinguish cases with strong and weak reasons for abortion. If proven and effective fetal therapies involving low morbidity and little risk to the mother existed for genetic disorders, the reasons supporting abortion would be less weighty. If, for example, treatment at the genetic or phenotypic level of a disorder were as effective as fetal blood exchange to prevent Rh isoimmunization, a strong moral argument against abortion could be made in those cases. No case of refused fetal therapy for Rh problems has been reported, to my knowledge. The point is that, ethically, treatment should follow diagnosis, unless another overriding moral reason can be given against treatment. If the potential for genetic treatment grows, parents and physicians will need to distinguish frequently between their legal right to use abortion and their ethical obligations to treat the fetus or newborn.

In reality, treatments for the vast majority of disorders that are prenatally diagnosable are either nonexistent or barely approximate a reasonable standard of efficacy. Shapiro reviewed treatments for genetic disorders (3). Therapy for genetic disorders is at present confined to the modification or palliation of the harmful expression of genes. An example is use of purified factor VIII for hemophilia A and von Willebrand's disease, both of which are prenatally diagnosable. The treatment is not totally effective or lasting; it is expensive and consumes an important resource. No genetic disorder is as yet treatable on the genetic level.

The effects on abortion choices posed by treatment can be illustrated by phenylketonuria. Treatment for PKU in newborns by a prolonged diet therapy was discussed in the first section. With techniques of DNA analysis, PKU is now prenatally diagnosable (75). Parents who have carefully treated an affected child with PKU now face a new choice in subsequent pregnancies, if they plan for more children. As they decide about prenatal diagnosis, ought the existence of a treatment that prevents serious mental retardation, albeit prolonged and distasteful, count heavily against the abortion option? Should potential harm of an abortion to the self-esteem of their treated child be a consideration? Will permitting abortion for a partially treated disorder dampen interest in developing better therapies? Such questions gain in significance as therapies for genetic disorders improve and as more persons who are at higher risk decide to have children.

The prevailing practice is to respect parental choices about abortion, including cases in which disorders are partly treatable. Parents will differ in their judgments depending upon previous experience and their ethical beliefs. But should such variability be permitted?

Writing earlier but in a relevant vein, Kass (57, pp. 196–198) objected to variable parental choice as the locus of genetic assessment for two reasons: 1) it conveyed the idea that children were the property of their parents, and 2) a hidden, natural standard of health and humanhood lay behind the appeal to parental autonomy, by which practitioners assess whether genotypes fall inside or outside true humanhood. Kass argued that such a natural standard was impossible to construct because of the great range of genetic variation. Without a clearly constructed objective standard, in his view, the variable reasoning involved in abortion choices could not logically be prevented from use to justify killing handicapped infants and older persons. Kass's points are worth review in the context of PKU cases.

Neither individual human beings nor nascent fetuses are property in the sense of a material possession to be bought and sold. Property is not the issue, however, but whether fetuses are persons entitled to societal protection *from* their parents in abortion choices. How much ought the interests of the fetus with a diagnosed disease count morally when in conflict with the interests of parents and family? A great deal depends upon physicians' abilities to treat the disease, as discussed above. Also, in a culture generally approving of parental autonomy in reproduction and abortion to the point of viability, conflicts could easily arise when the disease is treatable and yet the parents refuse treatment.

The case of PKU is a good example of this dilemma and a harbinger of things to come. In my view, moral policy on abortion choices for PKU (and other partially treatable disorders) ought to be to continue to support parents who make variable choices. The principle involved here is respect for parental autonomy about choices in reproduction and abortion. In effect, society has refused to take upon itself the task of elevating a genetically based natural standard to separate humans to be saved from abortion from nonhumans to be sacrificed to abortion. Such a standard cannot be constructed along empirically clear lines, as Kass saw clearly. However, society does permit parents to make assessments of the degree of genetic handicaps and nonpreventable suffering they can or cannot accept, without exacting a public accounting of their reasoning. The preferred approach to genetic abortion choices amounts to a rough *social* standard of intolerable suffering that relies upon the judgments of parents, using their own moral lights after expert counseling, to weigh the issue. This social approach, which tolerates diverse choices and outcomes, is not allowed after birth. I disagree with Kass (57: p. 197) that the standard to which "most physicians and genetic counselors appeal . . . no matter what they say or do about letting the parents choose" is a natural standard that separates the human from the nonhuman. Examination of the literature and participation as an observer in genetic centers shows that prevention of untreatable suffering is the major criterion used to justify genetic abortions. The actual standard is what kind of unavoidable suffering families can or cannot bear. The family's beliefs, its strengths and weaknesses, are what this society currently trusts in abortion choices rather than a category to separate what is human from nonhuman. The moral implication of Kass's argument is that in genetic abortion parents treat their rejected fetuses as nonhuman objects, or virtually as animals fit for slaughter. This characterization does not fit the reality of midtrimester abortion choices in any sense with which I am familiar. Quite to the contrary, parents suffer intensely from the burden of choice to end the lives of their own unborn offspring who are the victims of biological or environmental forces beyond their control or the ability of physicians to treat. Society currently invests these parents with the authority to choose life or death for the fetus, rather than authorizing a high genetic tribunal to separate the human from nonhuman.

When treatment possibilities improve, the strongest reason for abortion will be weakened. Whether society will continue to allow such variability when much better treatment alternatives are available is an open question. There will likely be, however, cases of parental refusals of proven fetal treatment for religious or cultural reasons. The options of toleration of their differences or coercion of such parents in these few cases need careful discussion in a new socially approved forum.

Moral policy for newborns with PKU ought to support active treatment, even if parents refuse therapy, although such a case has not been reported. In my view, one crucial and morally relevant difference distinguishes abortion choices and choices about treatment at other stages of life: the separateness of persons and the nonseparateness of the fetus. One can prevent the suffering of a newborn, who is separate from parents, who will not themselves be physically harmed even if their refusal is overruled. Finally, Kass's arguments are weakened by the lack of any empirical evidence that less interest has been shown in therapy for persons with genetic disease or for protection of handicapped persons because of toleration of parental variability about abortion choices. The culture is fortunately passive about arriving at moral consensus about who is or is not fit to live after birth, although it allows parents the option to avoid predictable suffering in the newborn if they choose.

Noninterference with parental choice is a public policy that avoids two worse alternatives, namely, the proscription of all abortions except those to save the life of the mother and the proscription of abortions in some diagnoses, including those that are borderline (47 XYY) or partly treatable (PKU). This approach would, however, move the locus of authority in genetic assessment to physicians' advice to legislatures as to which abortion choices should be proscribed. In such a situation, pregnancies would be socially guarded and tolerance for diverse choices would be suppressed.

PKU is also an instructive example for the future because it raises questions of the responsibilities of pregnant homozygous women, who have themselves been treated for PKU, who now carry fetuses for whom treatment may avoid serious harm. As more female children are successfully treated for PKU, their subsequent pregnancies are thought to have a better outcome if they observe the diet during pregnancy (76). What should be the attitude of physicians if such a woman is uncooperative in therapy? What is she refuses precautionary therapy? The ethics of abortion and the ethics of therapy, including therapy for the fetus with a genetic disorder, will surely continue to collide. My view is that a defensible moral line prevents any coercive or forced fetal therapy, even if it is proven, since pregnancy does not exempt physicians from the duty to obtain consent from the woman for any procedure that concerns the fetus (77).

Selective Feticide and Selective Birth in Twin Pregnancies

Cases arise in twin pregnancies in which one twin is diagnosed as having a disorder and the other is presumed normal. When this discordancy is known, parents have three choices: to continue to term with the higher risks of any twin pregnancy, to abort both twins, or to select feticide of the affected twin. In practice, the third option has been limited to centers with technical expertise to carry out twin diagnoses, methods of selective feticide that carry minimal risk for the healthy twin, and management of the continuing pregnancy to avoid the potential dangers of a dead fetus in the uterus, including clotting, hemorrhagic diasthesis, and shock.

In 1984, Antsaklis reviewed nine reports in the literature on selective feticide (78). The term "selective feticide" was first used by Rodeck et al. and is fitting because the dead fetus remains in the uterus to be delivered as a fetus papyraceous (79). The term "abortion" ought to be confined to acts that evacuate the uterus and are likely, but not certain, to cause fetal death. Some authors entitle their reports "selective birth" or "selective survival," and deny altogether the reality of the dead twin (78, 80). Both sides of the dilemma, as well as the medically relevant facts, include both terms "selective feticide" and "selective birth."

No follow-up study of parents who have made this difficult choice has been done, a serious deficit in accounting for the consequences of prenatal diagnosis.

Controversial Indications for Prenatal Diagnosis

When organized genetic services were first offered, indications for prenatal diagnosis were based upon serving well-defined categories in pregnancies known to be at higher genetic risk (53). These categories were agreed upon and utilized in admission of patients:

• women of 35 years of age or more
• a previous birth of a chromosomally abnormal child
• a parental chromosomal abnormality
• family history of chromosomal abnormality
• multiple (three or more) spontaneous abortions
• previous child with multiple malformations but no cytogenetic study performed
• pregnancies at risk for X-linked disorders
• pregnancies at risk for autosomal recessive disorders
• higher risk for neural tube defect

Today questions frequently arise whether prenatal diagnosis should be done apart from these criteria or on request by a pregnant women with a presentation of "anxiety." This problem is quite pressing in nations with a nationalized system of health care in which prenatal diagnosis is rationed. In Norway for example, amniocentesis is rationed and oversight given by a committee of Parliament (81). The maternal age cutoff in Norway is 38 years, and any provision to a younger woman, even though risks of chromosomal abnormalities are higher from age 35 to 37 than from age 33 to 35, is considered a serious breach of public policy. By contrast, in nations such as Switzerland and the United States, where market forces and consumer preferences play a large role in the health care system, far less control is exercised over the indications policy for prenatal diagnosis. For example, in Switzerland, of the 12,038 amniocenteses done between 1981 and 1983, 3,175 (26.4 percent) were for women under 35 for the indication of "anxiety" (82). Comparable statistics are not collected in the United States.

Maternal Anxiety

Should maternal anxiety be an indication for prenatal diagnosis? What is maternal anxiety? A definition is difficult since most pregnant women feel anxious about the potential for birth defects. Cases of maternal anxiety are difficult, especially in nations where prenatal diagnosis is rationed. In other nations, to give the procedure for anxiety begs the question of whether a trend is being encouraged to provide prenatal diagnosis for each pregnancy, if requested. Milunsky took this position in 1979 (83). Should society encourage a goal of providing genetic assessment in each pregnancy if the woman chooses? Such a goal is beneficial from a perspective of prevention, since in the United States and many other countries 75 to 80 percent of chromosomal abnormalities, including Down syndrome, will be found in children born to women under 35 years of age (84, 85). From the perspective of maximizing choice about reproduction and minimizing suffering, benefits would also follow. Seen in terms of equality of fetal interests, the trend would result in more abortions and be harmful.

Choices about prenatal diagnosis for maternal anxiety involve several complex factors. First, there are mental health considerations of the prospective patient and her family situation. Second, an existing policy of the nation or genetics unit about the lower limit on maternal age must be considered. Third, technical potential exists to diagnose Down syndrome in pregnancies of younger women by testing serum for evidence of lower values in alpha-fetoprotein, believed to correlate with the very low weight for age of the affected fetus (86).

Cases of maternal anxiety can be divided into three types: 1) cases of "morbid" anxiety related to preexisting mental illness or emotional problems that develop during pregnancy, 2) cases of "unfounded" maternal anxiety based on uproven risks of genetic harm, such as radiation exposure, cancer chemotherapy, and environmental exposure to mutagens (87), and 3) cases of "informed" maternal concern that may also involve anxiety based on knowledge of chromosomal risks or exclusion from access by existing policy on maternal age. Physicians are well-advised to seek psychiatric consultation before giving prenatal diagnosis in cases of the first type. In cases of unfounded suspicion of environmental harms, prenatal diagnosis should not be given, since no answer can be provided. Good arguments for lowering the maternal age cutoff to the early 30s have been endorsed by a President's Commission (7: p. 81).

Sex Choice Unrelated to Sex-Linked Disorder

Before DNA analysis provided a certain way to detect sex-linked disorders like muscular dystrophy and hemophilia in the fetus, couples were faced with a choice of aborting a normal male 50 percent of the time following disclosure of fetal sex after prenatal diagnosis. This unfortunate choice still faces couples wherever resources do not allow for development of these techniques.

Some couples who fall outside this group also want to know the sex of the child and intend to abort the fetus with unwanted gender. These cases divide into two types: 1) families with several children of the same gender, and 2) families from cultures with strong male preference (88, 89). Objections to sex choice have been made for reasons to conserve resources, protect against gender discrimination, and to avoid a backlash from those who oppose abortion (89, 90, 91). My own position against prenatal diagnosis for sex choice agrees with each of these reasons and adds a fourth. The problem of sex selection tends to reintroduce a feature of "positive" eugenics into contemporary medical genetics. Negative eugenics involves the prevention or amelioration of harms from genetic conditions. The genetic assessments made by parents described in this section fit this definition. Positive eugenics is an attempt to improve the species by enhancement of existing genes or deliberate selection of genotypes for reproduction deemed to be superior. Positive eugenics, in short, attempts to add a "plus" to the normal state. No genetic harm is involved in a family that has been unfortunate in the random assignment of gender at fertilization. To attempt to "treat" their disappointment by using prenatal diagnosis and abortion is harmful to the fetus and also may encourage ideas of deliberate preselection of gender. Since the sex ratio is virtually perfect, except in societies that systematically neglect female children at birth, change in the sex ratio is not needed. Sex selection involving methods prior to fertilization requires a separate discussion.

Problems in Disclosure of Diagnostic Results

In the view of most practitioners and parents, the goal of prenatal diagnosis is information about the presence or absence of disease in the fetus (8). Since diagnostic results are negative in more than 96 percent of cases, families are given many months of relief from anxiety. Also, contrary to past practice, many parents with higher genetic risks attempt to have children. Family disruption, divorce, stigmatization of parents, siblings, and other family members occurred frequently in high-risk groups (92). Pregnancies that would otherwise be aborted because of substantial recurrence risks can be safely carried to term after negative results are obtained. Because of the great moral significance of test results, medical geneticists are strongly committed to total disclosure. However, ethical conflicts sometimes arise that confront their commitment.

Disclosure of Fetal Sex

Chromosomal analysis reveals the sex of the fetus. Is there a duty to disclose fetal sex to parents, when it is not related to disease? Modell expressed concern about the practice of disclosing fetal sex in the context of first trimester diagnosis, which might create more opportunity for sex choice abortions (93). In the United States, no legal barrier to abortion for sex choice exists, although very strong ethical objections can be found to it. A physician could legally refuse to disclose fetal sex, since these data are incidental and not involved with disease. However, the practice is to disclose fetal sex to parents who want to know.

Disputed or Potentially Harmful Findings

Disputes can arise about the significance of laboratory findings (for example, true versus pseudo-mosaicism or the possibility of contamination by maternal cells (87: p. 17). When genuine doubt exists and too much time has elapsed to do a repeat procedure, what should the parents be told? Should conflict about findings and interpretation between professionals be revealed to parents?

Other difficult choices arise about disclosing information of probably small significance that will cause parents severe anxiety and may lead to psychological harm. One example is when sonography suggests an irregularity of the fetal head but the amniotic fluid is normal for alpha-fetoprotein. Some chromosomal findings that raise questions about the duty of full disclosure are 47 XYY and androgen insensitivity syndrome (XY females and XX males). Is the counselor obliged to disclose the history of controversy about criminality and XYY individuals? Will a full biological explanation harm the self-esteem of an individual discovered to have an opposite genotype from his or her sexual phenotype?

Cases of false paternity and also refusal of the patient to have information shared with relatives at higher risk also occur after prenatal diagnosis. The issues are virtually identical with those discussed in the previous section on genetic screening.

Problems in Access and Distribution of Services

Modell, among others, viewed access to and distribution of prenatal diagnosis as the central ethical problem in genetic assessment (93). She and others reported that in most developed nations less than 50 percent of women over 35 years of age have prenatal diagnosis, although about 80 percent request amniocentesis when informed about it (94). Except for Denmark, where about 80 percent of women with medical indications for prenatal diagnosis receive it, no nation meets the need for services in pregnancies at higher genetic risk. The best estimate of utilization in the United States is that probably no more than 10 percent of all pregnancies at known risk for genetic reasons are studied by prenatal diagnosis (53). Furthermore, women who undergo prenatal diagnosis belong largely to higher economic and social groups and are disproportionately white and urban (95, 96). Bowman (18) documented the economic and social barriers to services for black parents. Another factor limiting access is apparent underreferral by physicians (97). Lack of financial, technical, and human resources have restricted the distribution in many countries.

In the United States the problem of access and poor distribution of genetic services are aspects of the many inequalities that the society allows in the health care system. In terms of distributive justice, inequities in basic prenatal care have a higher ethical priority for correction than inequities in distribution of genetic services (98). However, policymakers must weigh the added burden to poorer and less well educated families and to society of lack of access to genetic services.

Ethical Guidance for Prenatal Diagnosis

On the basis of previous statements, practitioners and policymakers would likely agree with the following guidelines for prenatal diagnosis (7–9).

1.   Practitioners ought to safeguard, to the limits of their professional responsibilities, the range of choices open to parents after prenatal diagnosis, including abortion.

2.   Practitioners should serve parents who have ruled out an abortion option. Prenatal diagnosis should be provided when a valid indication exists or when parents need the information to prepare for the birth of a possibly affected child.

3.   Evidence related to risk and benefit persuades that the common practice of informing only women 35 years and older about prenatal diagnosis for age-related risk of chromosome anomalies in the fetus can be reevaluated to make diagnosis available to younger women.

4.   A request for prenatal diagnosis for maternal anxiety is an opportunity for counseling but by itself not a medically valid indication. Consideration of the indication of morbid anxiety should be done in consultation with a mental health specialist.

5.   Sex chromosome abnormalities (XO, XXY, XYY, and others) should be disclosed to parents following prenatal diagnosis, with a full description of the potential and problems of children and adults who live with these conditions.

6.   Androgen insensitivity syndrome (XY females and XX males) is a condition which should be disclosed to patients after chromosome studies. Special care should be taken to give an explanation that casts no

ambiguity on the patient's social and phenotypic sexual identity. A biological explanation must be given which includes the cause of infertility. The patient's level of education and knowledge are factors in how detailed the counselor becomes in the biological explanation.

7.   Parents should be asked in advance of prenatal diagnosis if they prefer disclosure of the sex of the fetus. When parents desire not to know in advance of delivery, practitioners should guard this information and alert the obstetrician and other relevant parties to the parents' preferences.

8.   Practitioners should not perform fetal diagnosis for sex selection alone, unrelated to a sex-linked disorder. Such requests are treated as appropriate for counseling, but not as a valid indication for prenatal diagnosis.

9.   Practitioners ought to provide special care to parents whose wanted pregnancies are terminated following genetic diagnosis to help them with loss and grief and avoid more complicated depressive states.

10.   Practitioners and society have duties to provide education and improve access for those who most need genetic services. Practitioners should also be active in education of the public about genetic services and the inequalities that exist in access to them.

Genetic Counseling

Genetic counseling has been defined by practitioners as "a communication process which deals with the human problems associated with the occurrence, or the risk of occurrence, of a genetic disorder in a family" (10). As defined by the statement, the goals of counseling are to help counselees: 1) to understand the medical facts, which include diagnosis, probable course of the disorder, and available management; 2) to learn about the way heredity contributes to the disorder, and the risk of recurrence in other relatives; 3) to know the options for dealing with the risk of recurrence; 4) to choose the course of action which seems appropriate to them in view of their risk and their family goals, and act in accordance with that decision; and 5) to make the best possible adjustment to the disorder in an affected family member or to the risk of recurrence of that disorder.

Genetic counseling involves value-laden choices and many conflicts of ethical duties, some of which have been described above and also in writings of practitioners and reports of interdisciplinary groups (99, 100). Perhaps the most significant ethical problem in genetic counseling arises from appeals by the counselee for moral direction, posed by questions like: "What would you do if you were in my place?" or "Do you have any advice for me?"

Nondirective or Directive Counseling

Most genetic counselors prefer nondirective counseling, out of respect for the ethical principle of autonomy and to safeguard the choices enjoyed in societies that practice noninterference with parental autonomy. In practice, nondirective counseling means that the counselor avoids giving specific moral advice or directives about which choice is "best." The counselor's strategy, as outlined by Applebaum and Firestein, is not to "present a counselee with our private agenda of interview content. We search for the counselee's agenda, and try to help the counselee achieve his or her objective by making available our knowledge of all facets and ramifications of genetic disorders" (101: p. 7). These counselors advise colleagues to "resist the temptation" to respond to appeals from counselees for moral guidance, explaining that "no outsider, professional or other, can do more than *imagine* what he would decide if placed in the counselees' shoes" (101: p. 8).

A report of an official ethics commission gave two reasons why most counselors prefer nondirectiveness (7). First, they want to disassociate themselves from an earlier period of eugenic beliefs and practices. Second, many nonphysicians entered the practice of genetic counseling and distinguished their role from the more familiar medical model in which the patient expected and received specific recommendations.

My view differs in part from that of Applebaum and Firestein. Appeals for moral guidance are not "temptations to be avoided," but opportunities for optimal counseling or referral for specialized help. The preferences of counselors notwithstanding, three realities of genetic counseling tend to cast doubt on whether nondirectiveness can be successfully practiced or is a completely satisfactory policy.

First, genetic counselors themselves have moral preferences that arise in each new case and become a part of the reality of the counseling situation. How can these preferences be denied? Counselors invite professional involvement in moral problems by defining their duties to help counselees evaluate their options and to make an appropriate choice. Such help presumably involves distinguishing between the technical and moral aspects of a choice. Counselors stress that their role in a moral problem is to help the counselee search his own or family's values and beliefs in making choices. However, once a professional enters into helping a client with moral choices, it is impossible to maintain the posture of a neutral and unbiased counselor. To present certain technical options, like prenatal diagnosis or sterilization, carries the assumption that the counselee would receive no moral blame in the context of the genetics center if she chose them. Hsia pointed to the "myth of the unbiased, nondirective counselor," and admitted that at most one could hope not to be "overly . . . or overtly directive" (102). Hsia also counseled counselors to be frank with counselees about their strong biases.

Second, counselees are often very interested in obtaining the benefits of the counselor's experience in how others have resolved the moral dilemma with which they struggle. Also, counselees rightly assume that counselors have experience in the moral aspects of human genetics that would benefit them. Scrupulous nondirectiveness deprives the counselee of valuable information. If the counselor emphasizes the counselee's authority to choose, the sharing of experiences about outcomes of struggles with moral problems is not being directive or manipulative, in my view. Surely, diversity will be the message. By describing diverse outcomes, the counselor gives an interpretation of the current moral situation. Society does not judge harshly a counselee's choices, as long as these are informed and voluntarily made. Another alternative is to ask counselees if they need help with the ethical aspects of their choice and to refer them to appropriate advisers. Counselees with strong religious ties may be in need of specialized help and instruction about the options available within their ethical traditions. A strict interpretation of nondirectiveness implies a "hands-off' policy regarding ethical issues. This is an unfortunate and suboptimal approach to counseling, which should be open to referral for mental health and ethical considerations that arise. If counselors jealously guard the task of helping counselees make choices, they may assume wrongly that the counselee should confer with no one else or that all clergy would be biased against the goals of genetic counseling. However, referral to reliable sources of information about moral traditions and pastoral counseling is being encouraged by genetic counselors (103).

The third reality is that counselees occasionally appear who are incompetent; examples are the mentally retarded parent or unemancipated minor. These clients require direction, especially when no close and involved family members are available to help chart a direction. Also, some counselees behave self-destructively and harmfully to the fetus, as in cases of drug or alcohol abuse. To maintain nondirectiveness may encourage more irresponsibility or lack of liaison with sources of help and change, such as mental health specialists.

Ethical Guidance for Genetic Counseling

With these caveats about nondirective counseling and on the basis of preexisting statements, practitioners and policymakers would probably agree with these guidelines for genetic counseling (7, 10, 11).

1. The most difficult choices in genetic counseling are ethical in nature, although such choices have medical aspects. For example, choices for donor insemination or abortion or sterilization involve ethical concepts of responsibility in parenthood and traditions of ethical guidance which are outside the special competence of the genetic counselor. While remaining sensitive to ethical aspects of such choices, genetic counselors ought to abstain from active or passive limitation of the autonomy of the individual whom they counsel. The principle of respect for the autonomy of counselees has the most universal acceptance by genetic counselors and is the most relevant resource for many conflicts in this field.

2. Genetic counselors ought to refer counselees to reliable sources of moral advice on request or offer referral when appropriate.

3. In counseling situations, adequate choices can be made only if the counselee is fully aware of the facts and features of the case. Genetic counselors should respect the right of the counselee to adequate and complete information.

4. The divulgence of data about the genetic condition of a counselee can adversely affect his or her personal and social welfare and the welfare of other family members. Genetic counselors should respect the highest standard of confidentiality in protecting information obtained in the course of their professional activities. These standards apply also to the handling of data and safeguarding personal genetic files.

Proposals for Ethical Guidelines for Familiar Problems in Genetic Assessment

Ethical guidelines for the most familiar problems in genetic screening, prenatal diagnosis, and counseling were posed at the end of each section. Although many practitioners involved in genetic assessment in the United States and Canada are trained genetic counselors or doctoral-level professionals, the great majority of medical geneticists in the world are physicians. Is there a consensus among medical geneticists on their approach to these problems? Would consensus be found in a cross-cultural perspective? This question is being studied in an international (19-nation) survey of more than 1,000 qualified medical geneticists (11, 104).

Is there a need for more expression about ethical consensus in medical genetics today? Three reasons support an affirmative answer, insofar as approaches to the familiar problems are concerned. First, medical geneticists deal daily with choices about human reproduction, an area of cultural life filled with strong emotions and laden with moral and ethical considerations. These problems call for skills and ethical sensitivities that exceed the demands of everyday medical practice. Some practitioners are not physicians. Valid questions can be raised about the ethical standards from which they proceed to genetic assessments. Parents and family members are entitled to know the ethical standards of the professionals who embark with them on weighty decision making. Policymakers also need to know the ethical standards of a specialty that is gaining in technical power to prevent and partially control genetic disorders in humans.

Second, although medical geneticists in many countries might agree to many, if not all, of the proposals above, their views remain in an "oral tradition" rather than in normative guidelines. A number of important documents and ethical discussions exist, but none represents the positions of official bodies of medical geneticists (5–10). Many medical specialties and subspecialties have clarified preferred approaches to the ethical problems that most frequently confront them. Medical geneticists can do likewise.

Third, and most important, the future of genetic assessment will be ethically far more complex if the questions raised below are indicative. From what ethical ground will medical geneticists face these issues? Facing them with the help of guidelines that consolidate and systematize what has been learned about moral experience to date is better than facing them simply with the strength of convictions.

Unfamiliar Ethical Issues in Genetic Assessment

The discussion has touched upon a number of unfamiliar and novel ethical issues in genetic assessment. These issues need further study and debate in a socially approved forum. Late in 1985 the U.S. Congress passed a law that established a Congressional Biomedical Ethics Board patterned after the Office of Technology Assessment (105). A 12-member board of six senators and six representatives, three from each party in each six-member delegation, will be supported by a 14-member Biomedical Ethics Advisory Committee representing various disciplines required for such efforts. The following issues need to be studied, debated, and recommendations published by the Biomedical Ethics Board.

Genetic Assessment

A time is foreseeable when much of the human genome will be mapped. What desirable and undesirable uses can be made of this knowledge? What are the ethical, social, and legal implications of virtually total knowledge of the contents of the human genome? What are the desirable limits of genetic knowledge about individuals and populations? What will advances in genetic knowledge mean in the practice of medicine, to the physician-patient relationship? What are the ethical principles that are most relevant to the developing issues in genetic assessment? How can these principles be used to separate desirable from undesirable consequences of greater genetic knowledge and more powerful techniques of genetic assessment? How should society prepare for the future of genetic assessment? What form of oversight, if any, is needed in this area of social life? Should it be a form of permanent public oversight as is practiced in Norway? Or is oversight of this field best left to practitioners working in a medical context?

Genetic Screening for Diseases of Later Onset

What are the ethical and legal issues involved in disclosure of a positive finding of a presymptomatic genetic disorder? Does it matter if the disorder is lethal and untreatable? What are the mental health considerations of such screening? What kind of supports do individuals and families need to cope with such knowledge? Should children or unemancipated minors be screened for such diseases? If minors are screened, what ethical constraints, if any, should be placed on disclosure of results? Do employers ever have a right to know the diagnosis? Do public safety considerations apply?

Genetic Screening for Susceptibility to Common Diseases

What are the social and medical benefits of screening tests for genetic susceptibility to common diseases? What are the ethical problems that could arise from such knowledge? How can those who are identified at highest risk be protected from forms of genetic discrimination in terms of opportunity for education, employment, and insurance? If such knowledge is attained, who should have access to it? How should such data be managed during the lifetime of the individual? Do employers ever have a right to know? Do public safety considerations apply? Do any age limits apply in such screening, and how should disclosure be conducted when and if children or unemancipated minors are involved?

Genetic Screening in the Workplace

What is the state of the art of genetic screening for susceptibility to hazards of the workplace? What protections for workers and employers are needed for research to develop and validate such tests? Assuming that such tests are reliable, should companies be permitted to select employees according to their genetic susceptibility for occupational illness? Should individual workers decide how to respond to the results of genetic testing themselves, or should employers control who is transferred? What protections for workers screened on the job are needed? What kind of consent process is needed for workers to be screened before employment?

Prenatal Diagnosis

What is the state of the art of prenatal diagnosis? Will a time arrive when it will be a desirable social goal for prenatal diagnosis to be available to any pregnant woman who desires it? If not, what are the boundaries of an effective and ethically sound indications policy for prenatal diagnosis? Should society consider placing limits on abortion choices following prenatal diagnosis? For example, if methods to determine severity of disease in the fetus are developed, should abortion choices ever be limited for the least severe and most treatable conditions? If treatments for genetic disorders become proven and effective, should abortion choices ever be limited for those disorders?

Treatment for Genetic Disorders

What is the state of the art of treatment for genetic disorders? Assuming that approaches to somatic cell gene therapy will be successful, would it be desirable to develop approaches to germline gene therapy? What desirable and undesirable consequences are posed by this option? Can effective moral lines be drawn and maintained between medical uses to prevent disease and eugenic uses of this form of genetic technology? If treatment at the genetic level in the fetus becomes proven, what approach should be taken to refusal of treatment? What approach should be taken today if a pregnant woman refuses proven fetal therapy? Does it make a difference if she has been successfully treated for a genetic disorder? Is forced or coerced treatment of a pregnant woman ever ethically justifiable?

Research in Genetics Involving the Human Embryo

Will diagnosis of chromosomal abnormalities or genetic disorders ever be feasible in the preimplantation human embryo? What scientific and medical benefits could be gained from such knowledge? What are the possible abuses of research with the human embryo? Should embryos ever be created for the sole purpose of research? Are laws necessary to protect the human embryo in research? Is there a relationship between an opportunity to diagnose genetic disease in the embryo and potential to treat? How does research in *in vitro* fertilization intersect with research possibilities for the earliest genetic assessment in the embryo? Should the recommendations of the Ethics Advisory Board in 1979 on federal support for research in *in vitro* fertilization be accepted or be restudied from the perspective of research bearing on genetic issues (106)?

Gametic Research

What is the state of the art of research into genetics in human gametes? Will it ever be possible to select gametes for fertilization to avoid harmful genes without doing harm to the gametes? What are the desirable and undesirable consequences of such research? Are new ethical considerations necessary for research with human gametes?

Sex Selection

What is the state of the art of predetermination of sex prior to fertilization? What are the desirable and undesirable consequences of sex selection? What are the social, ethical, and legal implications of preconceptual sex choice? Assuming that there will be effective and safe techniques to predetermine sex, should any limitation be placed on their use?

References

1. Rowley PT. Genetic screening: marvel or menace? Science 1984;225:138–43.
2. Ramsey P. Screening: an ethicist's view. In: Hilton B, Callahan D, Harris M, Condliffe P, Berkley B, eds, Ethical issues in human genetics. New York: Plenum, 1973, p 151.
3. Shapiro LJ. Treatment of genetic disorders. In: Emery AE, Rimoin DL, eds, Principles and practice of medical genetics. Edinburgh: Churchill Livingstone, 1983, pp 1488–1502.
4. Fletcher JC. Ethical considerations in and beyond experimental prospective clinical trials of human gene therapy. J Med Philos 1985;10:293–309.

5. Lappe M, Gustafson JM, Roblin R. Ethical and social issues in screening for genetic disease. N Engl J Med 1972;286:1129–32.
6. National Research Council. Genetic screening: programs, principles and research. Washington DC: National Academy of Sciences, 1975.
7. President's Commission for the Study of Ethical Problems in Medicine and Biomedical and Behavioral Research. Screening and counseling for genetic conditions. Washington DC: US Government Printing Office, 1983.
8. Powledge TM, Fletcher JC. Guidelines for the ethical, social, and legal issues in prenatal diagnosis. N Engl J Med 1979;300:168–72.
9. Fletcher JC, Hibbard B, Miller JR, Rudd N, Shaw MW. Ethical, legal and social considerations of prenatal diagnosis. In: Hamerton JL, Simpson NE, eds, Report of an international workshop, Prenat Diag (Special issue), Dec 1980, pp 43–46.
10. Ad Hoc Committee on Genetic Counseling. Genetic counseling. Am J Hum Genet 1975;27:240–42.
11. Fletcher JC, Berg K, Tranøy KE. Ethical aspects of medical genetics: a proposal for guidelines in genetic counseling, prenatal diagnosis and screening. Clin Genet 1985;27:199–205.
12. Merz B. Markers for disease genes open new era in diagnostic screening. JAMA 1985;254:3153–61.
13. McLaren A. Prenatal diagnosis before implantation: opportunities and problems. Prenat Diag 1985;5:85–90.
14. Warnock M. A question of life. The Warnock report on human fertilization and embryology. Oxford: Basil Blackwell, 1985.
15. Reilly P. Sickle cell anemia legislation. J Leg Med 1973;1:39–45.
16. Nalbaldian RM. Mass screening programs for sickle cell hemoglobin. JAMA 1972;221:500–2.
17. Jones SR, Binder RA, Donowho EM. Sudden death in sickle cell trait. N Engl J Med 1970;282:323–325.
18. Bowman JE. Mass screening for sickle hemoglobin: a sickle crisis. JAMA 1972;222:1650–51.
19. Whitten CF. Sickle cell programming: an imperiled promise. N Engl J Med 1973;288:213.
20. Goodman MJ, Goodman LE. The overselling of genetic anxiety. Hastings Cent Rep 1982;12:20–27.
21. Report of the Task Force on Genetic Diagnosis and Counseling. Genetic counseling, the church, and the law. St Louis: Pope John XXIII Medical-Moral Research and Education Center, 1979, pp 107–10.
22. Goffman E. Stigma: notes on the management of spoiled identity. Englewood Cliffs NJ: Prentice-Hall, 1963.
23. Kenen RH, Schmidt RM. Stigmatization of carrier status: social implications of heterozygote genetic screening programs. Am J Pub Health 1978;68:1116–20.
24. Massarik F, Kayback MM. Genetic disease control: a social psychological approach. Beverly Hills CA: Sage, 1981, p 103.
25. Stamatoyannopoulos G. Problems of screening and counseling in the hemoglobinopathies. In: Motulsky AG, Ebling J, eds, Birth defects: proceedings of the fourth international conference. Vienna: Excerpta Medica, 1974, pp 268–75.

26. Clow CL, Scriver CR. Knowledge about and attitudes toward genetic screening among high school students: the Tay-Sachs experience. Pediatrics 1977;59:86–91.
27. Childs B, Gordis L, Kayback MM, Kazazian HH. Tay-Sachs screening: social and psychological impact. Am J Hum Genet 1976;28:550–58.
28. Scriver CR, Bardanis M, Cartier L, Clow C, Lancaster GA, Ostrowsky JT. Beta-thalassemia disease prevention: genetic medicine applied. Am J Hum Genet 1984;36:1024–38.
29. Zeesman S, Clow C, Cartier L, Scriver CR. A private view of heterozygosity: eight year follow-up study on carriers of the Tay-Sachs gene detected by high school screening in Montreal. Am J Med Genet 1984;18:769–78.
30. Lappe M. The predictive power of the new genetics. Hastings Cent Rep 1984;14:18–21.
31. Gusella JF, Wexler NS, Conneally PM, et al. A polymorphic DNA marker genetically linked to Huntington's disease. Nature 1983;306:234–38.
32. Ray PN, Belfall B, Duff C, et al. Cloning of the breakpoint of an X;21 translocation associated with Duchenne muscular dystrophy. Nature 1985;318:672–75.
33. Knowlton RC, Cohen-Haguenauer O, Van Cong N, et al. A polymorphic DNA marker linked to cystic fibrosis is located on chromosome 7. Nature 1985;318:380–82.
34. Lehrman MA, Schneider WJ, Sudhof TC, Brown MS, Goldstein JL, Russell DW. Mutation in LDL receptor: ALU-ALU recombination deletes exons encoding transmembrane and cytoplasmic domains. Science 1985;227:140–46.
35. Weinberg RA. A molecular basis of cancer. Sci Am 1983;249:125–35.
36. Fletcher JC. Ethical and social aspects of risk predictions. Clin Genet 1984;25:25–31.
37. Bird SJ. Presymptomatic testing for Huntington's disease. JAMA 1985;253:3286–91.
38. Office of Technology Assessment. The role of genetic testing in the prevention of occupational disease. Washington DC: US Government Printing Office, OTA-BA-194, April 1983.
39. Brieger H. Genetic bases of susceptibility and resistance to toxic agents. J Occup Med 1963;5:511–14.
40. Jenson WN. Hereditary and chemically induced anemia. Arch Environ Health 1962;5:212–16.
41. Stokinger HE, Mountain JT. Tests for hypersusceptibility to hemolytic chemicals. Arch Environ Health 1963;6:495–502.
42. Stokinger HE, Mountain JT. Progress in detecting the worker hypersusceptible to industrial chemicals. J Occup Med 1967;9:537–43.
43. Koch EH, Bohn H, Koch F. Mucoviscidosis. Stuttgart: Schattauer, 1964.
44. Buist AS, Sexton GJ, Azzam AM, Adams BE. Pulmonary function heterozygotes for alpha 1 antitrypsin deficiency: a case-control study. Am Rev Respir Dis 1979;120:759–66.
45. Vogel F, Motulsky AG. Human genetics: problems and approaches. Heidelberg: Springer-Verlag, 1979, p 537.
46. Omenn GS. Predictive identification of hypersusceptible individuals. J Occup Med 1982;24:364–74.

47. Omenn GS, Motulsky AF. Ecogenetics: genetic variation in susceptibility to environmental agents. In: Omenn GS, ed, Genetic issues in public health and medicine. Springfield IL: Thomas, 1978, pp 83–111.
48. Severo R. Screening of blacks by Dupont sharpens debate in gene tests. New York Times, Feb 4, 1980.
49. Murray TH. Warning: screening workers for genetic risks. Hastings Cent Rep 1983;13:5–8.
50. Murray TH. The social context of workplace screening. Hastings Cent Rep 1984;14:21–23.
51. Fletcher JC. Moral problems and ethical guidance in prenatal diagnosis: past, present, and future. In: Milunsky A, ed, Genetic disorders and the fetus, 2d ed. New York: Plenum, 1986, pp 819–859.
52. Brambati B, Simoni G, Fabro S, eds: Fetal diagnosis during the first trimester. New York: Marcel Dekker, 1986.
53. Angell RR, Aitken RJ, Van Look PFA, Lumsden MA, Templeton AA. Chromosome abnormalities in human embryos after in vitro fertilization. Nature 1983;303:336–38.
54. National Institute of Child Health and Human Development. Report of a Consensus Development Conference. Antenatal diagnosis. NIH Publication No 79-1973, 1979, p I-74.
55. Council on Science and Society. Report of a Working Party: human procreation. Oxford: Oxford U Press, 1984, p 3.
56. Harrison BW. Our right to choose. Boston: Beacon Press, 1983, pp 123, 131.
57. Kass LR. Implications of prenatal diagnosis for the human right to life. In: Hilton B, Callahan D, Harris M, Condliffe P, Berkley B, eds, Ethical issues in human genetics. New York: Plenum, 1973, pp 185–99.
58. Lejeune J. On the nature of man. Am J Hum Genet 1970;22:121–28.
59. Ramsey P. The ethics of a cottage industry in an age of community and research medicine. N Engl J Med 1971;284:700–6.
60. Callahan D. Abortion: law, choice and morality. London: MacMillan, 1970.
61. Englehardt HT. Bioethics and the process of embodiment. Persp Biol Med 1975;18:486–500.
62. Grobstein C. From chance to purpose. Reading MA: Addison-Wesley, 1981.
63. Birch C, Cobb J. The liberation of life. Cambridge, England: Cambridge U Press, 1984.
64. Blumberg BD, Golbus MS, Hanson KH. The psychological sequelae of abortion performed for a genetic indication. Am J Obstet Gynecol 1975;122:799–808.
65. Donnai P, Charles N, Harris N. Attitudes of patients after "genetic" termination of pregnancy. Br Med J 1981;282:622–24.
66. Leschot NJ, Verjaal M, Treffers PE. Therapeutic abortion on genetic indications: a detailed followup study of 20 patients. In: Verjaal M, Leschot JH, eds, On prenatal diagnosis. University of Amsterdam: Rodopi, 1982, pp 85–95.
67. Adler B, Kushnick T. Genetic counseling in prenatally diagnosed trisomy 18 and 21: psychological aspects. Pediatrics 1982;69:94–99.
68. Jones OW, Penn NE, Schucter S, et al. Parental response to mid-trimester therapeutic abortion following amniocentesis. Prenat Diag 1984;4:249–56.

69. de la Chappelle A. Sex chromosome abnormalities. In: Emery AH, Rimoin DL, eds, Principles and practice of medical genetics. Edinburgh: Churchill Livingstone, 1983, p 214.

70. Haering B. Medical ethics. Notre Dame IN: Fides, 1973, pp 109–11.

71. Ramsey P. Ethics at the edges of life. New Haven CT: Yale U Press, 1980, pp 212–14.

72. Chervenak FA, Farley MA, Walters L, et al. When is termination of pregnancy during the third trimester morally justified? N Engl J Med 1984;310:501–4.

73. Powars DR. Natural history of sickle cell disease—the first ten years. Sem Hematol 1975;12275–80.

74. Merz B. Geneticists ponder ethical implications of screening. JAMA 1985;254:3160.

75. Woo SLC, Lidsky SA, Guttler F, Chandra T, Robson KJH. Cloned human phenylalanine hydroxylase gene allows prenatal diagnosis and carrier detection of classical phenylketonuria. Nature 1983;306:151–55.

76. Levy HL, Waisbren SE. Effects of untreated maternal phenylketonuria and hyperphenylalaninemia on the fetus. N Engl J Med 1983;309:1269–74.

77. Fletcher JC. Drawing moral lines in fetal therapy. Clin Obstet Gynecol 1986;29:595–602.

78. Antsaklis A, Politis J, Karagiannopoulos C, et al. Selective survival of only the healthy fetus following prenatal diagnosis of thalassemia major in binovular twin gestation. Prenat Diag 1984;4:289–96.

79. Rodeck CH, Mibashan RS, Abramowicz J, et al. Selective feticide of the affected twin by fetoscopic air embolism. Prenat Diag 1982;2:189–94.

80. Kerenyi TD, Chitkara U. Selective birth in twin pregnancy with discordancy for Down's syndrome. N Engl J Med 1981;304:1525–27.

81. Committee on Social Affairs. Parliament of Norway. Report No 91, 1982–83, pp 11–12.

82. Swiss Society of Medical Genetics. Medizinische Genetik No 12, 1984, p 11.

83. Milunsky A, ed. Genetic disorders and the fetus. New York: Plenum, 1979, p. 627 (ed. note).

84. Adams MM, Erikson JD, Layde PM, Oakley GP. Down syndrome: recent trends in the United States. JAMA 1981;246:758–60.

85. Holmes LB. Genetic counseling for the older pregnant woman: new data and questions. N Engl J Med 1978;298:419–20.

86. Cuckle HS, Wald NJ, Lindenbaum RH. Maternal serum alpha-fetoprotein measurement: a screening test for Down syndrome. Lancet 1984;2:926–29.

87. Hamerton JL, Boue A, Cohen MM, et al. Chromosome disease. In: Hamerton JL, Simpson NE, eds, Report of an international workshop. Prenat Diag (Special issue), Dec 1980, p 16.

88. Dove GA, Blow C. Boy or girl: parental choice? Brit Med J 1979;2:1399–1400.

89. Kazazian HH. Prenatal diagnosis for sex choice. A medical view. Hastings Cent Rep 1980;10:17–18.

90. Milunsky A. Know your genes. Boston: Houghton Mifflin, 1977.

91. Lenzer G. Gender ethics. Hastings Cent Rep 1980;10:18–19.

92. Meyerowitz S, Lipkin M. Psychosocial aspects. In: Preventing embryonic, fetal and perinatal disease. Washington DC: US Government Printing Office, DHEW Publication No (NIH) 76-853, 1976.

93. Modell B. Some social implications of early fetal diagnosis. In: Brambati B, Simoni G, Fabro S, eds, Fetal diagnosis during the first trimester. New York: Marcel Dekker, 1986.

94. Modell B. Chorionic villus sampling: evaluating safety and efficacy. Lancet 1985;1:737–40.

95. Sokal DC, Byrd JR, Chen ATL. Prenatal chromosome diagnosis: racial and geographic variation for older women in Georgia. JAMA 1980;244:1355–57.

96. Adams MM, Finley S, Hansen H. Utilization of prenatal diagnosis in women ≥ 35 years, United States, 1977–1978. Am J Obstet Gynecol 1981;139:673–77.

97. Lippman-Hand A, Piper M. Prenatal diagnosis for the detection of Down syndrome: why are so few eligible women tested? Prenat Diag 1981;1:249–57.

98. President's Commission for the Study of Ethical Problems in Medicine and Biomedical and Behavioral Research. Securing access to health care. Washington DC: US Government Printing Office, 1983, pp 60–61.

99. Hsia YE, Hirschhorn K, Silverberg R, Godmilow L, eds. Counseling in genetics. New York: Alan R Liss, 1979.

100. Capron AM, Lappe M, Murray RF, Powledge TM, Twiss SB, Bergsma D, eds. Genetic counseling: facts, values and norms. New York: Alan R Liss, 1979.

101. Applebaum EG, Firestein SK. A genetic counseling casebook. New York: Free Press, 1983.

102. Hsia YE. The genetic counselor as information giver. In: Capron AM, Lappe M, Murray RF, Powledge TM, Twiss SB, Bergsma D, eds, Genetic counseling: facts, values and norms. New York: Alan R Liss, 1979, p 184.

103. Fletcher JC, Baumiller RC, Lipman EJ. Clergy support for families. In: Weiss JO, Bernhardt BA, Paul NW, eds, Genetic disorders and birth defects in families and society: toward interdisciplinary understanding. White Plains NY: March of Dimes Birth Defects Foundation, 1984, pp 136–44.

104. Fletcher JC, Wertz DC. Ethics and human genetics: a cross-cultural perspective. Springer-Verlag (in press).

105. Public Law 99-158.

106. Ethics Advisory Board of the US Department of Health, Education and Welfare. Conclusions: DHEW support of research involving in vitro fertilization and embryo transfer. May 4, 1979; also Federal Register 44:35,1979.

III

Intrauterine Period

4

Ethics and the Termination of Pregnancy: The Physician's Perspective

WILLIAM G. BARTHOLOME

One of the most disappointing aspects of the current dialogue about abortion is the unwillingness or inability of many participants to view the ethical questions from the perspective of those individuals actually facing the issues. We seem caught up in a complex, convoluted, and endless controversy over the standing, status, interests, welfare, rights, and even experience of the fetus (1). Over the course of the last decade women have attempted to articulate a woman's perspective on the set of ethical problems raised by pregnancy termination. This evolving body of literature has helped many to appreciate the uniqueness of the relationship between the developing fetus and the pregnant woman and to understand that the ethical questions involved are not amenable to simple solutions (2). In this chapter I outline what might be called a physician's perspective on the ethics of abortion. I will demonstrate 1) that from the perspective of the physician there is a wide range of abortion problems; 2) that physicians play a variety of roles with associated ethical duties regarding abortion services; 3) that a physician has a set of ethical obligations to patients that includes provision of services relating to sexuality and reproduction; 4) that physicians have important ethical rights in the provision of such services to their patients; and 5) that a physician's ethical responsibility to patients can include assisting them in obtaining or providing them a safe abortion.

Abortion as a Grim Option

One of the most basic contributions made by women to the abortion dialogue has been helping us physicians to understand that abortion involves a decision of one profoundly undesirable outcome over another undesirable outcome. Abortion is at best a necessary evil. In an ideal world no woman would have to experience and no physician would need to perform an abortion. As a pediatrician, I most frequently encounter the ethical questions involving abortion when one of my adolescent patients and I discover to our shock and dismay that she has become pregnant. For me this suggests that many of the adults involved with this young woman have failed to act appropriately as caring and responsible providers. This same aspect of the abortion decision is faced by other physicians: the internist providing care to the woman with a life-threatening chronic illness who discovers that the woman has become pregnant; the geneticist who, in the process of evaluating a family for a possible serious genetic disorder, discovers that a member of the extended family has become pregnant; the urologist who has performed a vasectomy and discovers that the patient's spouse has become pregnant; the obstetrician whose patient has become pregnant in spite of the intrauterine device; and others. The diagnosis of pregnancy in these and a multitude of other cases is not welcome news, but rather the discovery of a set of serious moral problems for the patient and the provider.

A related important distinction is that between wanting an abortion and wanting a safe abortion to be available should one ever be needed. Women do not want abortions and physicians do not want to do abortions. Women want to be able to obtain safe and competent abortions if they should ever be unfortunate enough to need one. Physicians want competent abortion services to be available to their patients should they ever need them, and they want physicians who provide abortion services to their patients to be able to do so competently and compassionately. Even in the situation in which a woman has decided to undergo an abortion and a physician has decided to perform the procedure, both woman and physician want the abortion only in the sense that it is the only way of achieving a return to the desired nonpregnant state. The woman and her physician have elected this grim option as the least undesirable course of action in responding to her unintended pregnancy.

The Wide Range of Abortion Problems

Another unfortunate aspect of the public dialogue regarding abortion has been the minimal attention given to the diversity of the ethical questions, problems, and issues that occur because abortion involves such a wide range of cases and contexts. Although it is not possible to address the ethical issues raised by the entire spectrum of cases, an awareness of the range of issues can lead to an awareness of the multiplicity of the ethical problems abortion poses for physicians.

Age of the Pregnant Woman

One of the most obvious variables in the abortion decision is the age of the woman. As a pediatrician, I am all too aware that adolescent pregnancy is a serious problem facing our society. America's adolescent pregnancy rate is the highest in the world and represents one-third of all abortions done in this country (3).

Abortion in this context raises a variety of significant ethical questions. In many of these cases the young woman has become pregnant as a result of sexual abuse, incest, or statutory rape. In others pregnancy has resulted from ignorance or misinformation about sexuality. Many of those who have studied the problem believe that inadequate education about sexuality and inadequate access to contraceptive information and services play a crucial role. Pregnancy can also be the result of inadequately addressed psychological problems, a form of "acting out" behavior. Even when pregnancy is sought by adolescents, serious questions remain about the socioeconomic injustices that lead adolescents to see having a baby as a "way out," a solution to the problems of poverty, discrimination, social isolation, and despair that confront them.

There are also serious ethical questions that relate to the adolescent's relationship to her parents. Although for many adolescents the support of parents can be invaluable, for others parental involvement can have profoundly negative consequences. Do adolescents have an ethical right to privacy that includes confidentiality in the provision of contraceptive services and abortion, if necessary? Or do parents have a need or right to be notified in the event such services are sought or rendered to a minor? Are parents obligated to provide or assist their children in obtaining information about sexuality, reproduction, contraception, and abortion? How can the legal concept of the "emancipated minor" be incorporated into our ethical thinking about the adolescent who needs contraceptive services?

In addition to the special social status of the adolescent, physicians frequently consider her age in assessing the physical and emotional consequences of adolescent pregnancy. The health-related costs of pregnancy in this age range are thought by many to be relevant in evaluating the ethical justifiability of abortion for at least some early adolescents. Pregnancy also has a wide range of serious social consequences for an adolescent, including disruption of schooling, social stigmatization, isolation, and forced marriage. Few communities have created and made available the wide range of support services required for adolescents to bear and parent children adequately.

My own position is that a pregnant adolescent should have access to all the resources that would make it possible for her to assess the hard choice facing her. A strict requirement for parental consent cannot be justified ethically since it would place in the hands of the parents the power to compel the adolescent either to terminate or to continue her pregnancy. I also believe that the adolescent (particularly the adolescent who is not living at home) has a prima facie right to privacy and confidentiality in the provision of contraceptive services and abortion. I disagree with those who would require notification of the family (4).

Age can also be a significant factor in pregnancy occurring at the end of a woman's reproductive years. Advanced maternal age significantly increases both the maternal morbidity associated with pregnancy and childbirth and the risk of a variety of fetal abnormalities such as Down syndrome.

Medical Condition of the Woman

If there is any point of consensus in the abortion debate, it may be that abortion can be justified ethically in the case in which continuation of a pregnancy constitutes a direct threat to the life of the woman. Classically such justification was based on the principle of "double effect": the intended effect (saving the life of the woman) was distinguished from the foreseen, but unintended effect (terminating the pregnancy). Most modern justifications of abortion to save the life of the woman have been based on the woman's right of self-defense (5). The assumption in this view for the physician is that the woman's right of self-defense against an innocent attacker can justify the physician's assisting her in her defense. Although this view has recently been criticized (6), I feel that what can justify the physician's action in such rare cases is his or her special relationship to the woman. As I will argue later, the obligations to her entailed by the physician-patient relationship are one of the most neglected aspects of the abortion debate.

The importance of the variable of the medical condition of the patient is that the primary duty of the physician to the patient is in a sense a function of the patient's need for the special knowledge and skills the physician brings to their relationship. Even though the case involving a threat to the woman's life is uncommon, in this situation a physician may have a prima facie obligation to perform an abortion. The ethical basis of this obligation would not be the woman's right of self-defense, but rather the physician's obligation to prevent a serious harm to the patient, to preserve her life.

This obligation to prevent harm or protect the patient from the harm that could be associated with pregnancy or bearing a child is the basis of the so-called "medical indications for terminating pregnancy." Strictly speaking, no medical diagnosis or condition justifies terminating a pregnancy. Therefore, abortion is never simply a medically indicated procedure. However, a serious medical condition that is likely to be worsened by pregnancy or childbearing can serve as an essential ingredient in justifying abortion. Obviously, the difficult aspect of this approach has to do with defining and quantifying the harm or danger to the woman. Does the mere presence of a condition that would be worsened by pregnancy constitute an adequate justification? Does an emotional or mental condition that is likely to be aggravated by pregnancy or childbearing constitute harm that should be prevented? What probability of harm must exist before it is taken into account? Clearly any pregnancy involves significant health burdens and involves measurable risks of serious morbidity and even mortality. It is also well documented that the morbidity and mortality of vacuum aspiration abortion prior to 12 weeks' gestation is significantly less than carrying a pregnancy to term. How is this difference in risk to be assessed in ethical thinking about abortion?

Another complex set of abortion problems is raised by the presence of medical conditions that compromise the capacity of the woman to participate in decision making. The complex ethical problems involved in proxy decision making are raised in such circumstances and are rendered even more difficult when the pregnancy poses no particular threat to the life or health of the woman. Conditions such as severe or profound mental retardation, severe mental illness, or even stable conditions associated with reduced consciousness can force this complex set of problems on physicians and families. How is refusal to consent to abortion services by a retarded or mentally ill woman to be addressed (7)? The primary loyalty of the physician in such circumstances should be to the needs of the woman. If the woman is totally unable to participate in decision making, proxy decision makers should attempt to pursue the best interests of the incompetent patient, recognizing that these individuals would have limited or absent capacity to parent and no desire or interest in procreation. In most of these cases there are also serious ethical questions about the circumstances surrounding conception. Pregnancy may arguably be said to have resulted from serious neglect of the woman's need for effective contraception.

The Duration of the Pregnancy

Although over 90 percent of all pregnancy terminations are undertaken prior to the twelfth week from the last menstrual period or prior to the tenth week after conception, the late or "second trimester" abortion poses new and difficult ethical problems. One of the basic differences between early and late abortions involves the methods required to terminate the pregnancy. Late abortions may involve techniques that induce labor, with greater risk to the woman; she must also undergo a "labor experience" and the physician and others must attend the delivery of the fetus. In other cases, late terminations will involve cervical dilation followed by the destruction of the fetus via dismemberment. Either procedure is in many respects more difficult for the woman and the physician undertaking the procedure than those employed in the first trimester.

The duration of the pregnancy also poses difficult ethical questions because of the greater maturity of the fetus and its temporal proximity to the status of the premature newborn. In fact the concept of viability, which has played such a key role in the legal approach to the question of abortion, has proved to be a major weakness in thinking about abortion. As Callahan points out in his recent article on technology and abortion, advances in neonatal care have already resulted in the dividing line of viability shifting from 28 to 24 weeks' gestation (8).

Advances in our ability to respond to increasingly immature infants raises another serious moral question about late abortions. Although raised most dramatically by the occasional survival (even if brief) of fetuses after late abortions, the issue is more fundamental. If the goal of abortion is termination of pregnancy, it is possible to distinguish between removing the fetus or discontinuing one's support of the fetus and killing it. As technological expertise improves and the ability to support more immature infants improves, this issue will become more than a theoretical distinction. If the defense of abortion depends on the right of the woman to autonomy, self-determination, and the right to discontinue support of the fetus through abortion, the later in pregnancy one undertakes abortion, the stronger the argument that the pregnancy should be extended to the point at which care of the fetus can be undertaken by others through the use of advancing technology.

Abortion in the Context of Prenatal Diagnosis

Although only a small fraction of induced abortions is undertaken following prenatal diagnosis, such cases raise complex and unique ethical problems. In fact, the entire context in which abortion takes place is shifted when abortion is undertaken following identification of a fetal abnormality. In the vast majority of abortion decisions, the woman and her physician are using abortion to avoid continuation of pregnancy and the associated burden and harm of pregnancy and childbearing. In the situation of prenatal diagnosis, abortion is sought to avoid the birth of a particular fetus because he or she would be born with a particular congenital defect. The abortion is sought not to avoid the burdens and risks of bearing and parenting any child, but to avoid the burdens and problems attendant on the birth of a child with a particular set of problems and needs. It is the condition of the fetus and the future for the child that are seen as relevant to the decision whether or not to continue the pregnancy, not that of the woman. In some sense, then, the woman and physician can be said to be considering the abortion for the "sake of the fetus" and to protect the family from the unique set of problems and burdens that may arise in rearing a child with special needs. Yet fetuses can be afflicted with a wide range of congenital defects each associated with varying degrees of disability. Which fetal conditions can be said to justify termination of the pregnancy? Does the extent of the future child's likely handicap determine the justifiability of termination? Does it make a difference ethically if the congenital illness is amenable to therapy? How serious or life-threatening does the anomaly need to be? Although we could argue that fetal conditions that are usually fatal in early life (anencephaly, Potter syndrome, hypoplastic left heart syndrome, the lethal trisomy syndromes, and others) or that involve unremitting severe and progressive deterioration (Tay-Sachs disease, Hurler syndrome, metachromatic leukodystrophy, and others) might be severe enough to justify termination for the sake of the fetus, the vast majority of fetuses who are aborted following prenatal diagnosis have conditions that would meet neither criterion.

Considerable controversy continues on such basic issues as the utilization of prenatal diagnostic technology and abortion to select the sex of offspring (9, 10). Although it is difficult to find arguments to support a woman's (couple's) decision to abort a fetus in the second trimester because of its sex, it is even more difficult to justify a physician's undertaking a second trimester abortion on this basis (with the possible exception of the prenatal diagnosis of X-linked congenital illness).

From the physician's perspective, it is difficult to justify aborting a fetus with a congenital illness unless the congenital defect is incompatible with extrauterine life, fatal, or so severe that it would preclude or severely distort the child's development. I would argue that expansion of the idea of preventing harm or protecting the woman from harm, to include preventing the woman and her family from the burden of caring for a child with any congenital illness, is a considerable and controversial broadening of the concept of harm.

Another ethical problem involved in pregnancy termination in the context of prenatal diagnosis is that the diagnosis of the fetal condition is frequently not established until late in the course of the pregnancy. New technology in this area such as chorionic villus sampling or early amniocentesis may make it possible to establish some diagnoses earlier in pregnancy. However, fetal abnormalities discovered by more widely utilized technologies such as ultrasound screening or alpha-fetoprotein screening will continue to force women and physicians to face the ethical problems involved in late or second trimester termination.

Antecedents, or the 'Context of the Pregnancy'

No contemporary moralist has contributed more than James Gustafson in helping us understand the importance of context in shaping the abortion problem (11). Often the problem of the unintended pregnancy arises in the context of an ongoing relationship in which a physician has been attempting to help a patient control her fertility. Often the physician has provided and the woman has used contraceptives in this attempt. For both, a pregnancy arising in this context is experienced as a result of contraceptive failure. The pregnancy has occurred in spite of best efforts on both parties. Also, as Gustafson points out, an unintended pregnancy is almost never a problem that affects only the woman and her physician. Both the physician and woman are not only individuals but also persons in relation to others, persons involved in the ongoing lives, hopes, and aspirations of others to whom a wide range of duties, obligations, and responsibilities may be owed.

The failure to see abortion as arising for the woman in the context of her life process, plans, aspirations, and goals is a frequent and recurring criticism of the current abortion debate. The decision of whether it is more right on balance to terminate or continue a pregnancy is what might be called a paradigm case in contextual ethics. A woman's decision to continue a pregnancy entails such a broad range of duties, obligations, and responsibilities to herself, to the fetus, the future child, her immediate and extended family, and others with whom she may be involved in ethically significant relationships that it is more accurately called a choice about how to live one's life.

One context that is widely regarded as ethically relevant in the abortion dialogue is that in which the woman has become pregnant by virtue of sexual violence: sexual abuse, incest, rape. Most physicians feel strongly that terminating a pregnancy in these circumstances is as justifiable as termination undertaken to protect the patient from a threat to her life or health (12). Physicians perceive the woman who conceives in this manner as a patient having special needs by virtue of the trauma (physical, emotional, mental, and others) she has been forced to endure. Their experience and knowledge of the health-related consequences of such trauma make physicians particularly sensitive to the specialness of this context.

Additionally, prior to the legalization of abortion, physicians were frequently faced with the difficult task of meeting the health care needs of women who had obtained illegal abortions. For many physicians the fact that women cannot obtain safe abortions without their expert and compassionate assistance is a critical feature of the abortion question. One chairman of obstetrics pointed out that the experience of having one of your patients die from infection induced by an illegal abortion after you have been unable to provide her a safe one has a dramatic effect on one's perspective on the ethics of abortion.

The Role of the Physician

The roles of physicians in abortion and the ethical duties that attend these roles vary widely. One of the more obvious role differences is that between physicians who have the knowledge and skills necessary to perform the surgical procedures and related services involved in terminating pregnancy and those who do not. Not all physicians have the duty to provide abortion services. As a pediatrician, my role-related duties in abortion concern primarily my being competent in providing the broad range of education, counseling, and contraceptive information and services that would prevent my patients from becoming pregnant. Physicians in family practice or internal medicine would have a duty to develop and maintain a similar set of skills in order to render competent health care in sexual and reproductive aspects of their patients' lives. As mentioned before, abortion may be evidence that important needs of women were not being addressed. If all women had access to comprehensive health care by physicians who were capable of providing the range of services needed to allow women to control their fertility effectively, the rate at which abortion is performed in our society would be significantly reduced. The primary care physician also has a duty to patients to be able to make available to them, through consultation and referral, physicians and facilities that are capable of delivering the broad range of services needed by women who are considering pregnancy termination.

The role and duties of the obstetrician/gynecologist in abortion include those skills outlined above, particularly since they are the primary health care providers to a large number of women in our society. In addition, some contraceptive methods—for example, the insertion of intrauterine devices and tubal ligation procedures—require the special expertise of the obstetrician/gynecologist. In addition, however, the physician has a duty to acquire the knowledge and skills required to perform a competent abortion, although the need for them may never arise.

A small fraction (estimated to be 10–15 percent) of obstetrician/gynecologists are morally opposed to abortion in almost all circumstances. What are the ethical duties of the physician who conscientiously objects to the provision of abortion services? I would argue that such a position imposes special duties on that physician: 1) to disclose this position to his or her patients; 2) to avoid the imposition of special burdens or risks to his or her patient which might result from such a position; and 3) to provide mechanisms for consultation or transfer of responsibility for providing medical care when a patient might desire or need services, such as pregnancy termination. As I will discuss below, a physician has a right to refuse to provide any particular health care service, but the ethical duty not to neglect or abandon a patient requires that when the exercise of this right conflicts with the desires or needs of the patient, provision must be made for the patient to have access to an alternative source of care.

Additional role-related duties have to do with respecting the woman's right of privacy and maintaining the confidentiality of the physician-patient relationship. Obviously issues involving sexuality and reproduction are areas of our lives in which the needs of privacy and confidentiality are basic. Fulfilling these role-related duties often requires the physician to protect actively the patient from others who might seek access to confidential information. An excellent example of this problem and the challenges it poses for the physician is the case of the adolescent who seeks contraceptive services or an abortion. Particularly when the adolescent is living at home and is dependent on her parents, the duty to the adolescent to maintain privacy and protect the confidentiality of their relationship may seem to conflict with other obligations of the physician to the family. In fact some have argued that a physician in such a situation has a duty to notify the family before providing the services. Parents may well feel that they have a need to know if their adolescent daughter is seeking such services. It may also be possible to argue that the adolescent might benefit from the involvement and support her parents could provide. However, neither the perceived need nor the possibility of benefit to the adolescent would justify a strict ethical duty of parent notification. A physician might well point out to an adolescent facing an unintended pregnancy that the decision to maintain confidentiality from her family virtually precludes the option of continuation of pregnancy since the parents must eventually become aware of the pregnancy because of the adolescent's appearance. He or she might also encourage the adolescent to allow the parents to be notified and involved in addressing the problem if such a course of action is believed likely to yield benefits to the adolescent. However, I would argue that the duty to maintain confidentiality in such a situation can be waived only by the informed consent of the adolescent.

A parallel problem exists in the case of the woman's spouse or the biological father of the fetus. Does the duty of the physician extend to protecting the privacy and confidentiality of the woman from her husband or the individual claiming to be the father, or both? As a husband and father, I have considerable sympathy for a man in such a situation wanting or feeling a need to know that his spouse is considering terminating a pregnancy. I could also understand a spouse's desire to provide support and assistance to the woman who is undergoing an abortion. It may even be the case that a woman has an ethical obligation to notify her spouse that she is considering or plans to terminate "their" pregnancy. However, none of these needs, desires, or obligations can override the physician's duty to the woman to maintain confidentiality. Clearly, the woman has a critical need and a right to control the flow of information in such situations.

Other role-related duties may be due to the woman facing the problem of an unintended pregnancy. Such duties might include the provision of supportive counseling where needed, the provision of follow-up care to ensure adequate knowledge and availability of contraception, the provision of sterilization procedures where desired, and others.

The Physician-Patient Relationship

A central focus in the evolution of medical ethics has been the set of ethical obligations owed by physicians to their patients. Such obligations arise not from the role of physician but from the fact that individual physicians enter into and seek to maintain interpersonal relationships. The set of ethical obligations includes those owed by any individual involved in an ongoing relationship, such as the obligations to tell the truth, to keep one's promises, to avoid harm, and to provide help. In addition the special physician-patient relationship involves another set of obligations by virtue of the unique purposes and goals of such a relationship. These additional obligations can be based on and supported by an implicit and explicit contract between patient and health care provider or by the concept of a fiduciary relationship or convenant. They include such obligations as respecting the autonomy of the patient;

disclosing all relevant information regarding the patient's condition, treatment, and alternative treatments; preventing harm; providing necessary care; minimizing pain and discomfort.

Obviously many of these obligations are involved in the situation of a patient considering an abortion. I would like to begin with a clarification regarding what is sometimes referred to as "abortion on demand." The implication here is that the physician is ethically obligated to provide an abortion when such treatment is desired or demanded by a woman. Such an argument results from a misunderstanding of a physician's obligations in the abortion context. The informed consent of the woman to the termination of her pregnancy is a strict ethical obligation. It can be argued that performing an abortion without the woman's consent is prima facie unethical. However, a woman's willingness to consent to termination of her pregnancy does not logically or ethically oblige a physician to provide such treatment. An abortion-on-demand position profoundly undermines the moral status of the physician. It treats the physician as a provider of technical services, an amoral technician. Consent of the woman is an essential aspect of ethical decision making, but it is not itself sufficient to justify termination of the pregnancy. The physician is obligated to share in and carefully consider the abortion decision. In addition, the physician must be able to see his or her decision to perform an abortion for each individual patient as ethically justifiable. One of the most controversial and ethically problematic patterns of the provision of abortion services is the abortion clinic. Physicians in such clinics perform 15 to 25 abortions per day and have minimal involvement with the woman prior to or following the actual abortion procedure. In this situation physician and patient encounter each other as strangers. The physician has no way of knowing how the provision of abortion services fits into this woman's life plan, why the woman has chosen to terminate her pregnancy, how adequate counseling has been, and a host of other ethically significant factors. Physicians in such settings seem to have abdicated their ethical obligations with the exception of the actual provision of a surgical procedure in a safe and compassionate manner. At the very least, such an institutionalized pattern of health care raises serious ethical questions.

Aside from the obligation to respect the autonomy of the woman by obtaining her informed consent, physicians have other obligations to women considering pregnancy termination. One such obligation is a thorough discussion and exploration of alternatives to terminating the pregnancy. The woman may be seeking an abortion not because she considers it to be the most right (or least wrong) option but because she feels that she has no choice, no viable alternative given her present level of resources and obligations. Women facing unintended pregnancies are also vulnerable to coercion by others (spouses, family members, friends). In such a situation, the woman's decision is clearly neither voluntary nor autonomous.

The physician's obligation to prevent or protect the patient from harm is frequently an important ethical consideration. In fact, as I argued previously, this prima facie obligation can become a physician's actual obligation in the situation in which a pregnancy constitutes a direct, immediate, and serious threat to the woman's life. The exact nature of this obligation will vary with the type of harm threatening the woman. A woman's life can be in immediate jeopardy or threatened by serious harm that is virtually certain to occur if the pregnancy is allowed to continue. The harm can be one involving a serious temporary or permanent disability rather than a threat to life or maybe the exacerbation or relapse of a preexisting illness or the worsening or complicating of a chronic disease. These factors can be ethically relevant to the decision of the woman and her physician. However, I contend that none of these situations, with the possible exceptions of the loss of life or permanent disability, constitutes a sufficient justification in and of itself for the termination of a pregnancy.

Another important obligation of the physician relating to abortion is the provision of comprehensive follow-up services following termination. One aspect of this care is the obligation to provide the woman with the knowledge, counseling, and services that increase her ability to exercise effective and responsible fertility control. If abortion is a paradigm case of a grim option decision, it places an obligation on the woman to avoid as much as possible, the situation arising again. Since many of the most effective methods of control of fertility require the knowledge, skills, and services of physicians, a comparable obligation is placed on the physician.

A question might appropriately be raised about the physician's obligations to the fetus. I have used "obligation" to refer to ethically relevant features or characteristics of interpersonal relationships. Since the personhood of the fetus is clearly a point of significant and perhaps endless controversy, I hesitate to use the word "obligation" to talk about what the physician might owe the fetus (13, 14). However, as Feinberg has argued (15), fetuses are clearly the kinds of beings who can be said to have interests. For example, it can be argued that the fetus has an interest in not being harmed either deliberately or through neglect of its welfare assuming it will be born. In other words, if a woman is pregnant and chooses to continue to nurture the fetus and eventually to bear a child, she is obligated to respect the interest, entitlement, and right of the fetus not to be deliberately or negligently harmed. The physician is obligated to provide the knowledge, skills, and services that the woman requires to fulfill this obligation. In addition, the physician is obligated to avoid and prevent harm to the fetus in the context of a continuing pregnancy. However, as Feinberg points out, this interest of the fetus and corresponding obligations of the mother and physician to avoid and protect it from harm do not entail either logically or ethically a fetal interest in or right to be born.

Additionally, it may well be the case that at the stage of pregnancy at which a fetus is no longer dependent on the woman for its survival—so-called "viability"—the physician may well have strict obligations to the fetus. It may even be appropriate to talk about the fetus at this stage as a patient whose interests and rights can conflict with those of the physician's primary patient. At such a point in the development of the fetus, it may even be possible to argue that a physician is obligated to respect the fetus's interest in or right to be born, particularly if he or she can do so without significant harm to the interests or rights of the woman. However, even at this stage in the pregnancy, significant moral ambiguity remains as in cases of what has been called "forced cesarean section" (16).

The Rights of the Physician in the Provision of Abortion Services

One of the more underappreciated aspects of the Supreme Court's decision in *Roe v. Wade* (17) was that it vindicated the rights of physicians no less than those of women. In fact, as Tribe pointed out in his original review of the decision (18), the most fundamental aspect of this ruling was its "allocation of roles" in decision making regarding abortion. The court ruled that the most constitutionally defensible allocation of roles in this case was one that protected the rights of the woman and her physician to decide whether or not to terminate a pregnancy (at least prior to the state's interest at the "point of viability"). Thus, what is protected is both the woman's legal right to obtain an abortion free of state interference and the physician's legal right to provide such treatment according to his or her professional judgment. The court recognized a physician's right to make professional judgments and provide this form of medical treatment.

The ethical argument for a physician's right to perform abortions would be based on principles such as the physician's autonomy or liberty to practice his or her profession; the physician's duty to protect the privacy and confidentiality of the physician-patient relationship from state intrusion; the physician's obligation to prevent serious harm to the patient threatened by a pregnancy; and others. The most basic ethical argument would be that if the termination of a pregnancy were ever the actual ethical duty or obligation owed to a patient, the physician's right to perform such a procedure (without the threat of legal or other recriminations) is entailed both logically and ethically. Obviously a physician's right to perform abortions need not be unlimited, is at most a prima facie right, and does not mean it is always morally justified for a given physician to exercise that right in the care of a particular patient.

A physician may have other ethical rights in the abortion context. A partial list would include the right to refuse to provide abortion services (as long as such a refusal did not involve abandonment of the patient and such services were available from another physician); the right to refuse requests to disclose confidential information regarding abortion patients; the right to refuse to provide services to any particular patient (assuming that the procedure is "elective" and that there is no immediate threat to the life or health of the woman); the right to a fair compensation for services provided; and others.

The Ethical Responsibility of the Physician

Carol Gilligan in her provocative study of the ethical thinking of women facing the dilemma of an unintended pregnancy argues that women approach this moral problem not as a case of conflicting rights or principles, but rather in terms of the meaning and demands of the concept of responsibility (19). Many women see the ethical question as being the tension between acting selfishly and acting responsibly.

This feature of the woman's situation is the most basic ethical challenge facing a pregnant woman. As Martha Brandt Bolton reminds us, "respecting a fetus's right to be nurtured and developed involves a complex pattern of activities which form a prominent, demanding, and (in some cases) permanent part of one's life" (20). To continue a pregnancy a woman must assess the resources available to her in terms of a complex and broad range of responsibilities that would fall on her shoulders if she chose this course. These responsibilities—to her own health and even survival; to other persons who are dependent on her; to others to whom she may have ethical duties and obligations (for example, those of a lawyer); to nurture the fetus; to follow a demanding regimen of diet, exercise, health care, and the like; to avoid a broad range of activities that could place the developing fetus at risk; to carry, labor, deliver, and nurse an infant; plus the complex commitment of time, energy, emotion, and physical resources required to care for, to parent a child—are not necessarily logically entailed by the woman's decision to continue the pregnancy. However, given the nature of our society and the role-related responsibilities of women and mothers in it, careful consideration of these responsibilities is ethically demanded of the pregnant woman.

I would suggest that many physicians are not only aware of and sensitive to the role that the concept of responsibility plays in a woman's ethical reflection on abortion but utilize the concept in their own ethical thinking. A critical aspect of the ethics of the physician-patient relationship is that it involves a complex set of professional and personal responsibilities. To enter into and maintain such a relationship involves an open-ended commitment to a patient.

If the physician (involved in an established relationship with a patient) has accepted the responsibility of assisting a woman in the important task of controlling her fertility, an unintended pregnancy occurring in spite of their best efforts to control it confronts both woman and physician with serious questions of responsibility. This issue can be drawn in an even more demanding way if we examine the case of pregnancy occurring following the physician's performance of a sterilization procedure. In such a case the physician may have a prima facie obligation to provide an abortion if the woman involved was unable to assume the responsibility of nurturing the fetus and bearing a child.

I believe a similar argument involving the concepts of responsibility to provide care, responsibility for the health and welfare of the woman, and responsibility for one's actions and omissions could be used to examine a broad range of abortion problems. Does prevention or serious consideration of terminating the pregnancy fit into the set of responsibilities physicians owe women who are victims of sexual violence? Does a physician's responsibility to provide care to a woman for whom continuation of a pregnancy would entail serious risk to her physical or mental health include at least serious attention to the option of terminating the pregnancy? Does a physician's responsibility to a woman with severely limited competence due to mental illness who becomes pregnant without her knowledge or consent include serious consideration of abortion? If being a woman's physician involves accepting responsibility to meet that woman's health care needs in a competent, caring, and compassionate manner, there may well be a wide range of cases in which serious consideration of abortion will be ethically required. And there may well be some in which the physician can be said to have at least a prima facie obligation to perform an abortion.

Summary

In this chapter I have attempted to examine the ethics of abortion from the perspective of the physician. Since abortion involves terminating pregnancy and thereby ending the life of a developing fetus, it is always an ethical judgment that involves a choice of one course of action that is felt to be "less wrong" than another: a situation involving "grim options" or what might well be called ethical tragedy. If this is the case, a fundamental ethical consideration in any analysis of the ethics of abortion involves prevention of the problem that places women and their physicians in this "no win" situation: accidental or unintended pregnancy. Women, physicians, and many others in our society must attend to this important moral enterprise.

Although all abortions involve the core ethical problem of terminating a pregnancy and ending the life of the fetus, there is a wide range of ethical problems facing women and physicians in responding to the problem of an unintended pregnancy. In this chapter I have briefly examined some ethically significant factors, issues, and questions that include the woman's age, her medical condition, the stage of her pregnancy, the condition of the fetus, and the context of the pregnancy. I then considered what might best be called an ethical topography of abortion from the physician's perspective, the role of the physician and its attendant duties, the physician-patient relationship and obligations entailed by it, the ethical rights of the physician, and the physician's ethical responsibility to the woman.

From the physician's perspective there is a complex set of ethical duties, obligations, and responsibilities owed to the woman considering terminating a pregnancy. There may well be situations in which termination of a pregnancy can be a physician's ethical duty.

In closing, I am keenly aware that the author of this chapter was once a fetus developing in a woman's belly. I *am*, in an important sense, because she was then both able and willing to nurture me. If she had not been, I would want her to have had available a competent, caring, and compassionate physician.

References

1. Bondeson WB, Engelhardt HT, Spicker SF, Winship DH, eds. Abortion and the status of the fetus. Dordrecht, Holland: D Riedel, 1983.
2. Segers MC. Abortion and the culture: toward a feminist perspective. In: Callahan S, Callahan D, eds, Abortion: understanding differences. New York: Plenum, 1984, pp 229–253.

3. Henshaw SK, et al. A portrait of American women who obtain abortions. Family Plan Persp 1985;17(2):90–96.
4. Ooms T. A family perspective on abortion. In: Callahan S, Callahan D, eds, Abortion: understanding differences. New York: Plenum, 1984, pp 81–109.
5. Thompson JJ. A defense of abortion. Philosophy Public Affairs 1971;1:57–71.
6. Davis N. Abortion and self-defense. Philosophy Public Affairs 1984; 13(3):175–207.
7. Mahowald M, Abernethy V. When a mentally ill woman refuses abortion. Hastings Cent Rep 1985;15(2):18–21.
8. Callahan D. How technology is reframing the abortion debate. Hastings Cent Rep 1986;16:33–39.
9. Leff DN. Boy or girl: now choice, not chance. Med World News, Dec 1975;45.
10. McCormick RA. How brave a new world? Garden City, NY: Doubleday, 1981.
11. Gustafson J. A protestant ethical approach. In: Batchelor E, ed, Abortion: the moral issues. New York: Pilgrim, 1982, pp 191–210.
12. Survey: American College of Obstetricians and Gynecologists fellows (1985). Am Coll Obstet Gynecol Newsletter 1985;29(9).
13. Solomon D. Philosophers on abortion. In: Manier E, Liu W, Solomon D, eds, Abortion: new directions for policy studies. Notre Dame IN: Notre Dame Press, 1977.
14. O'Donovan O. Again: who is a person? In: Channer JH, ed, Abortion and the sanctity of human life. Exeter UK: Paternoster Press, 1982.
15. Feinberg J. Is there a right to be born? In: Rachels J, ed, Understanding moral philosophy. Belmont CA: Wadsworth, 1976, pp 207–220.
16. Annas GJ. Forced cesareans: the most unkindest cut of all. Hastings Cent Rep 1982;12:3–5.
17. Roe v. Wade, 93 Supreme Court 705 (1973).
18. Tribe L. The Supreme Court 1972 term. Harvard Law Rev 1973;87:1.
19. Gilligan C. In a different voice: psychological theory and women's development. Cambridge MA: Harvard U Press, 1982.
20. Bolton MB. Responsible women and abortion decisions. In: O'Neill O, Ruddick W, eds, Having children. New York: Oxford U Press, 1979, pp 40–51.

5

Fetal Therapy: Ethical Considerations, Potential Conflicts

ALAN R. FLEISCHMAN and RUTH MACKLIN

Physicians and midwives responsible for the care of pregnant women have always been interested in the well-being of both the mother and the fetus. Going back to the early Greeks and Romans, who conceptualized the fetus as a homunculus, a miniature person living and growing within the uterus, there was a fascination with understanding the process of fetal growth and development. However, only in this century has the mystery of reproduction been open to scientific scrutiny and much of the mysticism of the process of embryologic and fetal development been clarified by scientific investigation (1).

The last few decades have seen the increased development of the ability to measure fetal activity and growth, visualize the fetus through ultrasound, and monitor the fetus through biophysical measures. Most recently, direct medical and surgical interventions on the fetus have been accomplished. With this growing expertise in the assessment of the fetus *in utero*, both generally and with respect to specific medical and anatomic abnormalities, the fetus has emerged as a patient (2, 3). This patient clearly cannot participate in decision making concerning its own care and treatment. Its wishes cannot ever have been expressed, and it is completely dependent upon others to determine its destiny.

Inquiry into ethical issues in medicine has devoted much attention to decision making for patients incapable of deciding for themselves. The onset of fetal intervention provides a new arena in which to focus a number of familiar bioethical concerns and at the same time raises several new and unique issues. Parents must act in the role of surrogate decision makers for the fetus, just as they do in the case of medical care for their infants and children. However, decisions by mothers concerning their fetuses involve more than a consideration of the best interests of their offspring. Such decisions are also likely to take into account the mother's interest in her own bodily integrity and physical well-being, since all therapeutic interventions for the fetus require direct maternal participation. A woman in this situation thus becomes a surrogate decision maker for her fetus, as well as an autonomous decision maker for herself.

Medical, legal, and philosophical writings have described the potential benefits and harms of this new area of fetal assessment, fetal therapy, and interventions for fetal well-being. The goal of fetal assessment is preventing or alleviating disease or offering early in pregnancy the potential to abort a fetus who would otherwise be born with a serious congenital abnormality. Prevention of fetal and neonatal disease can be accomplished through altering maternal behavior, treating the mother for an illness, treating the fetus indirectly by giving medication to the mother, or intervening directly to treat the fetus medically or surgically. The goal of preventing fetal and ultimate neonatal disease is generally viewed as beneficial.

Furthermore, the goal of fetal assessment and monitoring during labor and delivery in order to prevent fetal compromise and irreversible damage by early and rapid intervention including cesarean delivery is widely held to be of benefit to the infant and the family. It can also be seen as beneficial to society in preventing the birth of infants with handicaps and disabilities.

The risks of these well-meaning interventions must, nevertheless, be explored. Attempts to prevent disease may inflict pain and suffering on mother and fetus and place either or both at risk for an outcome worse than the disease that was to be prevented. And, perhaps most poignantly, actions that may directly benefit the fetus have the potential to place the mother at significantly increased risk (4). In most cases the woman will believe the reliability of the data concerning the assessments of her fetus, will respect the expertise of the physician, and will thus be willing to accept the added risk of morbidity or even mortality to herself in the interest of her unborn child. However, a woman may not believe the information or perhaps not trust the physician's assessment both in terms of the potential risks to her fetus of nonintervention and the potential benefits of the proposed treatment. And finally, a woman may just be unwilling to place herself at added risk, no matter how small others may deem it, in order possibly to help her fetus.

The physician who desires to protect and promote the best interests of both the woman and her fetus may be faced with a real conflict: a pregnant woman who does not wish to place herself at any added risk for the potential benefit of her fetus. This poses the dilemma of determining where the physician's primary responsibility ultimately rests. Which of the two patients warrants full loyalty, advocacy, and concern, and how should the physician resolve this conflict?

In this chapter, we will examine the ethical dilemmas raised by these new medical capabilities regarding the fetus. The central dilemma is the potential for maternal-fetal conflict. We will look at fetal assessments and therapies, examine the ethical dilemmas, and identify the possible conflicts that may arise among caregiver, woman, and fetus. We will also address the issue of maternal behaviors that can place the fetus at risk, such as use of tobacco, drugs, and alcohol and the problems posed by hazards in the workplace. We will limit our discussion to the viable fetus and the wanted previable fetus, leaving concerns about the ethical dilemmas of the unwanted fetus to other chapters within this book.

Although some have argued that advances in fetal therapy have significant implications for the abortion debate (3), we believe the consequences are more subtle (5). Those at one end of the abortion spectrum who hold that it is morally permissible to abort a perfectly normal fetus are unlikely to grant greater moral protection to the fetus because of the ability to transform a defective fetus into a normal one. Similarly, the position of those at the opposite end of the abortion spectrum will remain unchanged, since for them, even defective fetuses have a "right to life" and so to abort them for any reasons is morally wrong. Both of these groups would claim that the health of the fetus and the potential for therapeutic intervention are irrelevant to the abortion controversy.

However, a third group might alter their beliefs about abortion as a result of the prospects for fetal therapy. This group holds that only some abortions are morally permissible: those in which the fetus is abnormal. If fetal therapy holds out the promise of correcting some abnormalities, abortion in those cases would no longer be acceptable. Thus, nothing in these new developments alters the basic structure of the classic debate between pro-choice and pro-life forces. The only changes likely to occur are in those for whom the permissibility of abortion is conditional, depending on whether the fetus has defects.

Fetal Therapy

The field of fetal therapy, including fetal assessments, treatments, and interventions, can be divided into three areas: 1) treatment of the mother in order to assist the fetus, 2) direct medical and surgical treatments of the fetus, and 3) the use of cesarean delivery in order to enhance fetal outcome. In each of these areas, a number of different parties have potential interests: the pregnant woman, the father of the fetus, the fetus itself, physicians and other health care personnel, and perhaps the larger society.

Two leading principles of bioethics are applicable here. The first is known as "respect for persons." This principle incorporates two ethical convictions: that individuals should be treated as autonomous agents and that persons with diminished autonomy are entitled to protection (6). This principle supports the right of the woman to determine what happens to her body, including the fetus, which is undeniably a part of her body. The principle of respect for persons might also be viewed as granting the fetus protection because of its diminished autonomy, although this application of the principle is more controversial. It depends on whether a fetus is the type of entity that possesses autonomy, albeit diminished. According to this principle, the physician has a clear moral obligation to respect the autonomy of the mother and a somewhat less clear obligation to protect the fetus, with its diminished autonomy. Stated another way, the physician has an obligation to protect the wanted fetus because of its future potential for full autonomy.

The second relevant precept of bioethics is the principle of beneficence. Persons are treated in an ethical manner not only by respecting their decisions and protecting them from harm, but also by making efforts to secure their well-being (6). Beneficent actions, in this sense, are best expressed by the rule: Maximize possible benefits and minimize possible harms. The physician who acts according to this principle seeks to protect and promote the best interests of both the mother and the fetus. This requires an objective assessment of the various therapeutic options and the implementation of those that protect and promote the best interests of both patients. The outcome should secure the greatest balance of benefits over harm (7).

The principle of beneficence applies as well to the decisions and actions of the pregnant woman. She has a moral obligation to act in the best interest of her fetus, at least insofar as she has decided to allow the fetus to come to term as a wanted offspring. In this situation, the interests of the fetus do not stem from its moral status as an independent entity but derive from its future standing as an infant and child, a full member of the moral community.

We will examine the three areas of fetal therapy: maternal treatment, fetal treatment, and cesarean delivery for fetal well-being. The ethical analysis will call on these two principles of bioethics.

Maternal Treatment to Enhance Fetal Outcome

Treatment of the pregnant woman to enhance the outcome of pregnancy is not new. Maternal medical illness has long been known to have an adverse effect on fetal outcome. Treatment of the mother who suffers from diabetes, hypertension, obesity, thyroid disease, renal impairment, and other conditions can create an environment that optimizes fetal well-being. This type of intervention has clear benefit for both woman and fetus, enhancing the health of both and placing neither at increased risk.

Changes in the care of the diabetic woman who becomes pregnant have been used to represent some of the most beneficial approaches to perinatal medicine (8). It has been shown clearly that careful control of diabetes and maintenance of blood sugar in the normal range by diet and the use of multiple insulin doses per day during pregnancy can decrease the likelihood of stillbirth, fetal abnormalities, and disease in the newborn. This treatment has some benefit to the mother as well, since control of diabetes is helpful in maintaining a feeling of well-being, in addition to preventing long-term complications of diabetes.

This type of fetal therapy, which treats a maternal illness, would seem to create little conflict for the reasonable patient. There are, however, two potential areas of conflict. First, treatment requires a strong commitment by the pregnant woman to diet, monitoring of blood sugar, and compliance with a very specific therapeutic regimen. Many patients are unwilling to subject themselves to this amount of regulation even for their own health. Although the treatments are not risky, they do impose on the patient's time and personal freedom and may be rejected. Moreover, the careful control of diabetes during pregnancy has a much greater effect on fetal well-being than on maternal well-being. The patient who is compliant with a treatment regimen when not pregnant is required to be far more careful and compulsive in her care when she is pregnant. She may find it difficult to make this personal sacrifice for the potential benefit of her fetus.

A second serious potential conflict occurs in the case of a treatment that would clearly benefit both mother and fetus but is unacceptable to the mother because of her strongly held religious or moral beliefs. An example is the Jehovah's Witness who chooses to refuse blood transfusion while pregnant. If the pregnant woman was going into shock because of blood loss, it would be highly likely that the fetus would be directly damaged if the mother's blood volume was not restored. The strongly held religious belief, which most physicians would reluctantly honor in a woman who is not pregnant in accordance with the principle of respect for persons, becomes a much more difficult moral choice when the fetus will be damaged by the woman's refusal of treatment. A New Jersey court has taken the view that a Jehovah's Witness could be transfused over her objection because she was pregnant and would otherwise risk both herself and her fetus if the transfusion was not given (9).

These types of decisions place the physician in a potential conflict over the duty to respect the woman's autonomy and beneficence—the duty to act in the woman's best interests as well as the best interests of her fetus. Following the principle of beneficence, the physician would strive to maximize possible benefits for both patients. The two principles of bioethics yield conflicting duties in this situation. In the case cited above, the court ruled that it was in society's interest to override the woman's refusal, despite her strongly held beliefs.

Medical therapy for the fetus can also be administered by giving medication to the mother for direct fetal benefit without maternal benefit. Some of these medications do have the potential to add to maternal risk without any measurable maternal benefit. One example of this type of treatment is the use of adrenal steroids in premature labor to enhance fetal lung development and prevent respiratory distress syndrome after the infant's premature birth. The steroid hormones have been shown to decrease neonatal mortality and morbidity, but at the same time to increase the risk of a postpartum infection in the mother (10).

Other examples of this type of fetal therapy include the *in utero* treatment of genetically determined biochemical defects (11). Many inborn errors of metabolism can now be diagnosed *in utero* through analysis of amniotic fluid obtained by amniocentesis. It has been shown that early treatment after birth enhances the outcome of many of these disorders. It is postulated that for some disorders, treatment *in utero* would result in even better long-term outcome. One such defect is methylmalonic acidemia. Some of the patients afflicted with this complex metabolic disorder benefit by the use of large doses of vitamin B_{12}. The earlier this treatment is initiated, the more likely there will be a good long-term outcome in terms of survival and central nervous system function in the baby. It has been reported that high doses of B_{12} have been given to one pregnant woman carrying a fetus with this disorder, with a good outcome (12). This vitamin supplementation adds no known risks to the woman while benefiting the fetus. Other vitamin-responsive inborn errors of metabolism might similarly be benefited by antenatal treatment.

A more problematic group of fetal patients treated by administering medication to the mother are fetuses with cardiac arrhythmias (13). Drugs such as digoxin, verapamil, propranolol, procainamide, and quinidine have been used in an attempt to regulate fetal heart rhythms when abnormalities seriously jeopardize fetal well-being. These drugs, when given in adequate dosage to assist the fetus, can affect the mother.

Complications of the mother's heart function and rhythm may occur, and uterine tone and contraction may be altered by these medications, thus affecting labor and delivery. These treatments have become standard in major tertiary centers capable of carefully monitoring both the fetus and the mother. Benefit to the fetus is substantial if the arrhythmia can be controlled, but potential risk to the mother is significant.

As more treatments are developed for the fetus that have little, if any, benefit for the mother but place her at increased risk, the possibility of maternal-fetal conflicts increases. Not only does this pose a problem for making risk-benefit assessments, it also leads to the tendency to view the fetus as an independent patient with the woman relegated to the status of little more than a maternal environment.

Direct Fetal Treatment

Medical and surgical therapeutic interventions can be administered directly to the fetus. These therapies include the injection of materials directly into the fetus or the amniotic fluid, as well as surgical attempts at correction of fetal abnormalities. Although these treatments are given directly to the fetus, they require inserting needles and instruments through the woman's abdominal wall and uterus in order to reach the fetus. All fetal interventions, no matter how direct, invade the body of the woman and increase her risk of various complications of the procedure.

Perhaps the best example of this group of treatments is intrauterine transfusion of blood into the abdominal cavity of the fetus who has severe anemia secondary to Rh sensitization (14). This technique, developed in the early 1960s, has succeeded in preserving the lives and enhancing the outcome of fetuses who would otherwise have died *in utero* of severe Rh incompatibility, or would have been severely impaired and who were too early in gestation to be viable outside of the uterus (15).

Potential conflicts include the mother refusing this invasion of her body, as well as refusing the blood transfusion of the fetus because of strongly held religious or moral beliefs. We are not aware of such a case coming to legal adjudication, but the weighing of the competing interests in analyzing the risks and benefits of this complicated treatment of a previable fetus would certainly be a difficult exercise for the court.

In recent years there has been a great deal of enthusiasm about the prospects of treating fetal congenital abnormalities surgically *in utero*. Three specific disorders have received much of the attention: obstructive hydrocephalus (16), bilateral hydronephrosis (17), and diaphragmatic hernia (18). Many fetal abnormalities can now be detected before birth with careful use of ultrasonography. Because many, if not most, pregnant women are having ultrasound examinations early in pregnancy to assess fetal size and gestational age, there is an increasing incidence of the early diagnosis of fetal abnormalities. Most of these abnormalities are best treated after birth, but prenatal diagnosis can serve the additional purpose of helping to prepare the family and medical team for the necessary treatments after delivery. For a fetal abnormality to be a candidate for *in utero* surgical intervention, it must meet the following conditions: it would have to be a relatively simple structural defect that directly affects organ development; the organ development would worsen over time if the defect were not corrected; and if the defect were alleviated the organ development would proceed normally or be less impaired than otherwise (19).

Experimental surgery for obstructive hydrocephalus has been performed on singleton fetuses less than 32 weeks' gestation with no other detectable, significant abnormalities, and whose ventricles were progressively enlarging, causing thinning of the cortical mantle of the brain. This disorder is extremely complex, and its course *in utero* is unpredictable. Hydrocephalus may progress to destroy virtually all of the brain cortex *in utero;* or, unpredictably, it might not progress and can stabilize. Furthermore, the cause of the hydrocephalus is rarely clear *in utero.* It may be associated with an underlying brain abnormality that will not be benefited by correction of the hydrocephalus. It also may be part of a more generalized complex of congenital malformations. In the reported studies, even with the most careful evaluation, 28 percent of the cases had anomalies found at the time of delivery that had not been detected *in utero* (16). To date there have been no randomized controlled studies to support the efficacy of this surgical intervention, and the entire procedure remains experimental. This group of patients poses a troubling ethical dilemma stemming from the prospect of a worse outcome after treatment than if no treatment had been administered at all. *In utero* surgery offers the potential to salvage a fetus who otherwise would have died of the abnormality, but who survives with profound brain damage and no ability to develop neurologically or cognitively.

The second fetal abnormality that has received surgical attention is urinary tract obstruction. Urinary tract obstruction *in utero* has two serious developmental effects on the fetus. First, the obstruction may result in dilatation of the renal tract and backup of urine, causing significant damage to the developing kidney. Second, the fetal urine excreted *in utero* into the amniotic fluid is necessary for normal lung development *in utero.* Absence of adequate amniotic fluid results in underdeveloped or hypoplastic lungs. Alleviation of the obstruction of the renal outflow tract can reverse or decrease the ultimate damage to the kidneys. However, restoration of normal amniotic fluid volume may not result in adequate lung development. Success depends upon the severity of the developmental disorder that has occurred and the time in gestation when the amniotic fluid is restored. Thus, irreversible renal damage, irreversible lung damage, or both may have already occurred when the fetus is diagnosed as having this abnormality. Here, again, the most difficult problem is being able to select just which fetus might benefit from the proposed treatment. This is a separate concern from those of the obvious potential risks of the intervention itself to the fetus and, to a lesser extent, to the mother.

The third fetal congenital anomaly that has been considered for surgical intervention is diaphragmatic hernia (18). In this disorder a defect in the diaphragm results in the abdominal contents herniating into the chest *in utero*. Surgical correction of the defect is relatively easy after birth, but even with successful surgery and excellent neonatal management over 50 percent of the infants die due to pulmonary insufficiency. The infants are unable to be ventilated due to pulmonary hypoplasia caused by compression of lungs secondary to the herniated viscera in the chest.

Appropriate candidates for *in utero* treatment of this disorder are fetuses with hypoplastic lungs that would develop sufficiently after decompression to support extrauterine ventilation better than would be the case if surgery were delayed until after delivery. There is little enthusiasm at the present time for *in utero* therapy of this group of patients because of the difficulty of identifying appropriate candidates.

We have spent some time describing the three most common fetal surgical interventions that have been proposed in order to clarify the complexity of these disorders and the difficulty in making assessments. Surgical intervention is not as straightforward as one might think, not only because of the technical difficulties of operating on a small fetus *in utero*, but also because of the developmental problems of the organs associated with the anatomic defects. A great deal of information is still lacking about which patients will benefit from the interventions, and among these, much is unknown about all of the concomitant risks. An international registry of all *in utero* surgery has been proposed and exists for voluntary reporting of cases in order to increase and centralize the information (19).

The fact that fetal surgical interventions are still in the experimental stage is uncontroversial. Because this fetal therapy is experimental, it calls for an ethical analysis different from that appropriate for established therapies involving the same group of interested parties—the pregnant woman, the fetus, the father, the physician, and other health professionals. We believe that any physician who wishes to proceed with a research maneuver has an obligation to seek advance review and approval of the research by an appropriate committee designated for that purpose. Such committees, known as Institutional Review Boards (IRBs), are required in every institution in the United States that receives funds from the Department of Health and Human Services (DHHS) for biomedical and behavioral research on human subjects. Officially required only to review research conducted or funded by DHHS, most of which is sponsored by the National Institutes of Health (NIH), these committees are now in place virtually everywhere in this country (20). Most IRBs, at least those in academic medical centers, review all research projects conducted in their institutions, whether or not they are funded in whole or in part by grants from the NIH.

Federal regulations governing the conduct of research on human subjects charge IRBs with two main tasks. The first is to review the risk-benefit ratio of proposed research projects to ensure that the benefits outweigh the risks. While the risks of human experimentation are always borne by the subjects, the potential benefits are calculated to include others besides the research subjects themselves—future sufferers from the same condition. In the case of experimental fetal therapy, although the fetus is the target of the research maneuver, the mother is also directly affected, so the risks to her must also be included in the risk-benefit calculation.

The second task of the IRB is to determine that the requirements are met for obtaining voluntary, informed consent from research subjects or from their legally authorized representatives, in the case of those unable to grant consent for themselves. This typically involves a careful review of the proposed consent form, but rarely includes monitoring the actual process of gaining informed consent from patients, or in the case of infants and children, from their parents or guardians. Review by the IRB thus serves to protect subjects by ensuring that the information provided (at least on the written consent form) about the purpose of the research, the procedures to be used, the risks, benefits, and alternatives, is complete and understandable to a layperson. However, the IRB is much less able to make sure that the other aspect of informed consent is present: that consent is granted freely, without any duress or coercion of the patient or surrogate.

As with any other experimental intervention, parents are not obligated to grant consent on behalf of their fetus for in utero therapy. Physicians recommending fetal therapy must disclose all of the uncertainties surrounding the procedure and potential outcomes, especially the prospect of an outcome worse than leaving the disorder untreated. A feature of any experimental procedure, particularly one in the early stages of development, is that the precise risks and benefits are unknown. Insufficient data from previous trials makes it difficult to calculate the risk-benefit ratio for the fetus alone; and the additional risk to the mother must also be taken into account. In the face of all these risks and uncertainties, parents should be allowed complete latitude to decide as they see fit. Even urging them to decide in their fetus's best interests is problematic, since that is one of the unknown factors.

Still another complicating issue may emerge: What if the parents disagree about whether or not the experimental therapy should be undertaken? This same question might arise about any proposed research on children for which parents must grant consent. And, for that matter, it could arise in cases of nonexperimental treatments for minors. Ironically, perhaps, the problem of parental disagreement is easier to resolve in the case of experimental in utero therapy than in these other cases. This is because the woman must grant consent for herself, as well as for her fetus. Her consent or refusal to consent becomes the overriding consideration, owing to the principle of respect for persons. If no fetal therapy were involved, a husband could surely not grant or refuse consent for a procedure on his wife, so long as she was competent to decide for herself. As long as the woman's body is invaded, placing her at some risk, however small, her choice about in utero therapy must be decisive.

Cesarean Delivery for Fetal Distress

The most troubling aspect of fetal intervention is the potential conflict created when a pregnant woman in labor refuses to consent to a cesarean delivery recommended by her physician because of impending fetal distress. This situation has arisen in recent years because of the development of techniques in fetal monitoring during labor, enabling the physician to assess fetal well-being better during the process of labor and delivery. This aspect is most troubling for two reasons. First, the techniques of fetal monitoring are by now well established, and while their predictive power is not perfect, they cannot be considered experimental or still in the research phase. Second, and more important, the advanced stage of fetal life suggests that the fetus has a greater moral standing at this point. The fetus about to become an infant is still unquestionably a fetus, given its direct physical dependence on the mother. Yet the question of whether its interests should be construed more like those of a neonate than a fetus is critical for the attempt to resolve the conflict posed by the mother's refusal of cesarean delivery.

Fetal monitoring, which includes the continuous measurement of fetal heart rate and rhythm as well as uterine contraction, is accomplished externally by a belt placed around the woman's abdomen or internally by an electrode placed on the scalp of the fetus to monitor the fetal heart and a catheter placed in the uterus to monitor contractions. These continuous measurements have been in use for over 25 years. They have resulted in careful analysis and the ability to determine patterns of heart rate and uterine contraction, which serve to predict risks for the development of acidosis, asphyxia, and ultimate hypoxic-ischemic encephalopathy or irreversible brain damage. Techniques have also been developed to sample fetal blood in utero by pricking the scalp through the dilated cervix to ascertain fetal acid-base status and thus increase the data upon which prediction is based about ultimate fetal outcome.

These assessment tools have been developed with the laudable aim of seeking to prevent fetal and ultimate neonatal compromise, resulting in the birth of normal newborns. The inevitable consequence of more careful fetal assessment has been an increase in the number of cesarean deliveries recommended for fetal distress. Suggestions to clinicians on how to use the data are biased in support of cesarean delivery to prevent fetal compromise before it is irreversible. Therefore, a significant percentage of fetuses are born by cesarean delivery although they do not require it, and would suffer no irreversible damage if delivered vaginally. The quality of the assessment tools at present does not allow separation of this group of "false-positive" candidates for cesarean birth from the "true-positive."

A development of another sort over the last 10 years has been the dramatic increase in medical malpractice suits against obstetricians for the birth of brain-damaged babies. With the decrease in the number of pregnancies per family, unrealistic expectations about the ability of technology to predict bad outcomes and a seeming general intolerance of a less-than-perfect offspring, our society has experienced a concomitant increase in lawsuits. Many of these suits result in awards to the plaintiff of millions of dollars. A general consequence has been a significant increase in medical malpractice insurance premiums. Thus, physicians, aware of this potential outcome if the fetus is irreversibly damaged, are recommending even more cesarean deliveries to protect the fetus from damage and to protect themselves from criticism and possible liability for not doing everything for the fetus to prevent damage.

This is the background against which the pregnant woman must make a decision when her physician recommends cesarean delivery. She may realize the fallibility of the data the physician has used to make the recommendation and she probably knows that cesarean delivery rates have risen to almost 30 percent of all deliveries in large university teaching hospitals. She is appropriately reluctant to place herself at a fourfold increased risk of dying during childbirth in addition to the significant pain and potential morbidity of the operation. She also may be told that the cesarean delivery can adversely affect her future reproductive life, making rupture of her uterus in pregnancy more likely and repeat cesarean delivery for each future birth far more probable.

This complex weighing of the competing issues is typically performed at the time of active labor. The woman is lying in bed, in at least intermittent pain and probably constant discomfort. She is attached to an intravenous infusion, a fetal monitor, and perhaps other devices. She may have received medication for pain relief, which can affect her ability to analyze alternatives. This situation results in the woman not being able to make a clear, rational, and informed decision. Most frequently, she respects the advice of her physician and concurs with the proposed plan presented as the best course for her baby. The atypical woman who questions the certainty of the data, voices concerns about her own well-being, or raises a question about the motivation of the physician concerning future malpractice protection, is viewed as a difficult, noncompliant patient who wishes to hurt her baby.

Another group of mothers refuses cesarean delivery based on strongly held religious or moral grounds. These patients believe that surgery under any circumstances is unacceptable. For them, surgery to protect the fetus is no more acceptable than any other medical technological intervention. These patients often do not come to the hospital for their deliveries and choose to deliver at home instead. However, some desire to be hospitalized but will not consent to surgery or other specific treatments. This group of patients has the same concerns as the former group of patients, and in addition, they harbor a general mistrust of the values, goals, and actions of the medical profession. They are far less subject to persuasion, explanation, or to being convinced of the appropriateness of the recommended surgery.

The general view that women who refuse cesarean delivery are in some way willfully abusing their fetuses is prevalent, at least among some physicians and judges (21). This results in physicians seeking court intervention to force a woman to undergo a cesarean birth for fetal well-being. The 1973 landmark decision of the Supreme Court, *Roe v. Wade*, recognized the right of a woman to obtain an abortion up to the point of fetal viability. It went on to hold that the individual states may create laws that limit abortion after the time of viability. This has been interpreted to mean that the state has a compelling interest in protecting the life and health of the fetus after viability (21). But the state does not have such an interest if the life or health of the mother is endangered by carrying the child to term.

Two very important court cases in this area are analyzed in an article by Robertson (9). The 1964 New Jersey case, *Raleigh-Fitkin-Paul Morgan Memorial Hospital v. Anderson,* involved a hospital petitioning to transfuse a Jehovah's Witness who was eight months' pregnant and in danger of a severe hemorrhage that would result in the death of her fetus and probably herself. The trial court held in favor of the woman's refusal, but the New Jersey Supreme Court ruled that the unborn child was entitled to the law's protection, and ordered the blood transfusion. Seventeen years later in 1981, and eight years after *Roe v. Wade,* the Georgia Supreme Court, in the case of *Jefferson v. Griffin Spalding County Hospital Authority,* ordered a cesarean delivery for a woman in her 39th week of pregnancy for both maternal and fetal reasons due to the diagnosis of a complete placenta previa. The court based its decision on the grounds that "the intrusion invoked into the life of [the mother] is outweighed by the duty of the State to protect a living, unborn human being from meeting his or her death before being given the opportunity to live."

In a similar case in Colorado, the court in ordering a cesarean delivery over the woman's refusal went so far as to describe the risk to the woman of cesarean delivery under general anesthesia as not so great as to preclude the state from preferring the interests of the fetus and ordering surgery (4). The legal analysis in these cases relies on value concepts and ethical argument. The next section describes two ethical frameworks in which such judgments can be made.

Ethical Analysis

Although not an entirely novel issue, the situation in which two patients have possibly competing interests arises out of the recent capability to deliver therapy directly to the fetus in utero. It may be instructive to recall other examples of potential conflict, old as well as new. The birthing process itself posed ethical dilemmas long before the advent of modern technology. The classic form of that dilemma is: When a choice must be made between the life of the baby and the life of the mother during childbirth, which should be saved? It is safe to generalize that opinion has been overwhelmingly in favor of preserving the life of the mother in these anguishing cases. But unlike the situation of fetal therapy, in which the pregnant woman must grant informed consent, it is probably true that in those classic cases, the women themselves were not participants in the decision to save their babies at the expense of their own lives.

In recent years organ transplantation using an organ from a live, related donor has provided another example. In this situation, one perfectly healthy person is rendered a patient by volunteering to donate a paired organ, tissue, or bone marrow to a relative in need. Following a medical assessment, and a judgment that the potential benefits to the recipient outweigh the risks to the donor, the relative is asked to grant consent to donate the organ. As in the case of the woman asked to grant consent for therapy on her fetus or to undergo a cesarean delivery for the sake of her infant, the voluntariness of the consent is seriously compromised. Can persons with a close relative in end-stage renal failure ever be said to give consent for removal of their own kidneys in a free or uncoerced manner?

Even if they cannot, an ethical defense of the practice can still be provided. When the donor and recipient are related, the donor is under an obligation to act in a beneficent manner. That obligation is stronger for persons who are related than it is for strangers or mere acquaintances. Similarly, the bond of kinship between parent and child—in particular, mother and newborn—carries with it moral obligations as well as deep human emotions. Altruism stemming from kinship may be partly rooted in biology, but it also forms the basis for the social structure of families in modern times as well as historically (22). Thus there is a natural tendency for people to act in a beneficent, even a self-sacrificing manner toward close relatives, a tendency reinforced by a set of role obligations that family members have toward one another.

The unique relationship of mother and child also stems from extremely high expectations for the offspring in an era in which families have fewer children. As the number of children decreases, the importance of each child increases. The fetus and newborn infant are often considered direct extensions of the mother and can be seen as the product of a desire for immortality (23). Thus, although bioethical analysis generally has dealt with the complex problem of the risk to one person for the benefit of another in the medical context, the specific ethical analysis of potential conflicts between mother and fetus relies on more basic biological, cultural, and psychological bonds between the two patients. This complicates the ethical analysis by enlarging the duties owed by the mother to her fetus.

Bioethics provides two contrasting approaches for conducting an ethical analysis of potential maternal-fetal conflicts. These two frameworks for ethical analysis are a rights-based approach and a consequentialist approach (24). It is not uncommon in analyzing a problematic issue in applied ethics to appeal to the rights of interested parties and also to the consequences of deciding or acting one way rather than another. Discussions of fetal therapy sometimes argue the rights of the woman in whose body the fetus is lodged in opposition to the rights of the fetus as an independent entity having interests. At the same time these discussions address the balancing of risks and benefits and the difficulties that arise when much uncertainty surrounds the calculation of risks and benefits. It is not clear in advance which approach to the analysis, rights-based or weighing of risks and benefits, will be superior in clarifying this complex area; however, the ethical issues may remain hopelessly unresolved if the two frameworks for analysis are conflated.

The problems that arise if the issue of fetal therapy is addressed from a perspective of rights are simple to enumerate but complex to resolve. Is the fetus properly considered a bearer of rights? In order to answer that question is it necessary to determine or to decide whether or not the fetus is a person? If the fetus is accorded the status of a patient, does that automatically imply that the fetus is to be considered a person that is a full bearer of rights? If there is an increasing acceptance that the already born neonate has rights, does the fetus who will become a neonate have all of the rights attributed to the already born? There are already firmly established rights of women in the reproductive area. How do the emerging discussions of fetal rights affect the rights of the woman? If the fetus and mother both can properly be said to have rights, what ought to be done when these rights come into conflict with one another, and how can these conflicts of rights be adjudicated? Must an advocate be appointed for the fetus in cases of conflict, and if so, what ought to be the characteristics or qualifications of such an advocate? And, finally, what role in the decision and what rights, if any, should be accorded the father of the fetus and/or the husband of the woman in cases where the fetus and woman are in conflict?

Some of these rights questions have been addressed in the context of the abortion controversy. Whether the fetus is properly considered a bearer of rights is central to the ongoing abortion debate. So, too, is the question of the personhood of the fetus, these two questions often going hand-in-hand. To adopt the position that the fetus is not a person but merely becoming a person does not automatically settle the question of rights because even nonhuman persons, such as animals, may be the bearers of certain rights.

Some have argued that elevating the status of the fetus to a patient automatically implies that the fetus is a full bearer of rights. Feminist writings have lamented the fact that the fetus is now being construed as a patient. One article observes that "it is clear that at this point pregnancy has become a disease with two potential patients—the pregnant woman and her fetus—and of those, the fetus is medically and technically by far the more interesting one." The pregnant woman is being referred to "as though she were merely the container in which the real patient—the fetus—gets moved about" (25). The concern of the author quoted is that once construed as a patient, the fetus acquires rights to medical intervention, rights that may override those of the mother in the eyes of physicians and judges. The author explicitly notes: "In this way the fetus's presumed 'rights' as a patient can be used to control pregnant women."

This argument points out a common problem in using a rights-based ethical analysis. One's antecedent position on a moral issue often determines whether an entire class of individuals should be the bearer of certain rights. There is often no clear antecedent basis for claiming that a class of individuals has those rights other than the claimant's desire to bring about a better state of affairs (26). We believe that in struggling with the ethical issues surrounding fetal therapy, it is not a helpful tactic to ascribe rights to the fetus and then try to effect a balancing act with the rights of the mother. In the legal domain, there may well be no other alternative than to attempt to balance rights when they come in conflict, but in the moral sphere, where questions of rights are much less settled, a debate resting on rights claims will reach either a stalemate or a rhetorical pitch.

An alternative approach is to bypass the problematic talk of fetal rights and of personhood and refer, instead, to the interests of the parties involved. This forms the basis of a consequentialist approach, in which the right course of action is the one that maximizes good consequences. In medical contexts, this perspective takes the form of an analysis in terms of risks and benefits. Construed somewhat more broadly, consequences can be viewed along utilitarian lines, embodying much more than simply the risks and benefits of treatment for the parties concerned. Even if approached in the narrower framework, though, the risks and benefits that need to be taken into account include those that accrue to the pregnant woman as well as to the fetus. The risks to both parties should not be minimized in the eagerness to describe the potential benefits to one.

As familiar as the consequentialist approach is to clinicians and researchers in medicine, this approach is not without its problems. The difficulty of predicting outcomes can be formidable. It can also be overlooked or minimized by physicians eager to offer benefits to their patients. Despite the enthusiasm with which the possibilities of fetal therapy have been embraced, as well as the arrogance in using fetal assessments during labor as absolute predictors of fetal distress and bad outcome, it must be emphasized that the diagnostic and therapeutic procedures applied to the fetus involve significant risks to the fetus itself. There is great difficulty, particularly in the area of fetal therapy, in making accurate risk-benefit assessments. This is always a problem in innovative diagnostic and therapeutic interventions, but it is heightened in the case of the fetus because of the increased uncertainties. This is true of direct medical and surgical therapy on the fetus as well as for the problem of recommending cesarean delivery for fetal distress.

The uncertainty about outcomes is only one problematic feature of a consequentialist approach to the ethics of fetal therapy. Not only do the risks to the fetus need to be balanced against the potential benefits, but also the risks to the mother must be taken into account at the very least by way of balancing them against the risks to the fetus of nontreatment.

There is yet a further difficulty, apart from the considerations that make it difficult to do the balancing of risks and benefits. The ultimate decision maker, the woman, is not a neutral party, toting up risks and benefits for all who stand to be affected by the action. The decision maker must be the woman on whom an invasive procedure will be performed for the sake of her unborn child. In most cases the mother will see her own interests as identical with those of the fetus, but this is not a foregone conclusion. The use of the utilitarian model for analysis suggests the need for a "neutral" outside decision maker. This notion is rejected by those who hold that patient and family autonomy should prevail in almost all circumstances in the medical sphere. At least some, however, would argue that an "advocate" should be appointed for the fetus (27). Some researchers have suggested that "it is best if a separate advocate can be identified for the fetus. This person not only seeks the best treatment for the fetus but also protects it from unwarranted or unnecessary assaults. Being separate from the fetus and the parents, the advocate can more objectively view the entire situation and the potential interventions. In some cases the advocate may recommend no intervention and thus relieve potential parental guilt" (27).

This proposal gives rise to several concerns. What would occur if the advocate for the fetus disagreed with both parental and clinical recommendations concerning in utero therapy? If parents are thought to do what is best for their infant and are prepared to go along with physicians' recommendations for treatment, why would it be necessary or desirable to involve an outside decision maker? Should the advocate be allowed to override or second-guess the physician and family who are in favor of treatment? How might the disinterested advocate be in a better position to ascertain what is in the best interests of the fetus than the other parties involved? The strategy of invoking the "disinterested observer" or advocate is often used in areas of great uncertainty because of the difficulty of decision making, and the fear of the subjective bias on the part of those most closely involved. But it is implausible to think that the advocate will be any better at making the difficult decisions than the involved parties or that the advocate, because of lack of emotional involvement, will be any more objective in weighing the various risks and benefits. Those involved in making decisions in matters of uncertainty must accept the weighty responsibility and deal with the complex emotions generated by these difficult decisions.

In other areas of biomedical ethics, committees have been instituted for assisting in making recommendations in cases of similar uncertainty and complexity. These multidisciplinary groups, composed of disinterested parties, should be invoked only to review and recommend when physicians and families, having already come to some thoughtful conclusions based on risk-benefit analysis and considerations of best interest, have reached no agreement (28). Rather than appointing an advocate for the fetus, we believe it would be more appropriate here, as elsewhere in biomedical decision making, to use an ethics committee to assist in making recommendations in difficult cases and to enhance "ethical comfort" for both the families and the treating physicians.

In our opinion, one great advantage of using a consequentialist approach for ethical analysis of fetal interventions is that it is less likely to make mother and fetus adversaries in battles over their respective rights. To pit the rights of the mother against those of the fetus is a divisive tactic, which has the prospect of heightening the difficulties rather than enhancing and promoting harmony in an effort to arrive at the best outcome for all concerned.

Maternal Behaviors

We have so far examined the ethical dilemmas generated by the need to make decisions concerning fetal diagnostic and therapeutic intervention. Another group of ethical concerns relates to the effects on the fetus of various maternal behaviors during pregnancy. These issues include the environment in which the woman lives and works, as well as her personal habits: nutrition, alcohol and drug use, and smoking.

The horrors of World War II gave a graphic example of the impact of ionizing radiation on the growing fetus. Fetuses exposed to such radiation developed multiple congenital anomalies and subsequent medical disorders (29). Other similar toxic environmental hazards have been noted for many years. However, the first systematic observation of a specific pattern of malformation secondary to maternal behavior was reported in 1973 when the fetal alcohol syndrome was described (30). Subsequently, therapeutic drugs and recreational substances, as well as smoking, have been clearly associated with fetal abnormalities (31). For each of the known teratogens there is a substantial risk to the fetus, but there remains uncertainty as to the extent of that risk. In the case of fetal alcohol syndrome, for instance, only 10 percent of infants show the stigmata when born to moderate drinkers who have continued to drink throughout pregnancy. Even for the heaviest of drinkers, only 60 to 70 percent of the offspring will be abnormal (31). Thus, although the risks are substantial, there is considerable predictive uncertainty about which infants will suffer the effects of maternal use of alcohol during pregnancy.

As in the case of fetal therapy, a consequentialist ethical analysis can be applied to maternal-fetal conflicts stemming from maternal behaviors that place the fetus at risk. The benefits to the mother include the pleasure and satisfaction she derives from the use of intoxicating substances. The risks of harm to the fetus and, for that matter, to her own health, weigh much more heavily, yielding a clear balance of risks over benefits by way of moral conclusion.

Care must be taken, however, to separate the health risks to the woman from the effects of her behavior on her fetus. In discussing the problem of maternal-fetal conflict, we can only properly include the risk of harm to the fetus in the risk-benefit equation. Although the self-inflicted harm to the woman is undeniable, at least in the examples of drug and tobacco use and excessive use of alcohol, those harms to self do not enter the picture of an ethical analysis of maternal-fetal conflict. The moral principle that governs disapproval of the woman's behavior and efforts that might be made to change it is the "harm principle": interference with a person's liberty can be justified in order to prevent harm to others. But to try to change the woman's health-risking behavior for her own sake is paternalistic. Whether or not medical paternalism can ever be justified is an important topic in its own right, but one that is not pertinent to our concerns in this chapter. We confine our analysis to the question of forcing the woman to comply with a healthful life-style for the sake of her fetus, a fetus who will become a child.

The question then becomes: Is application of the harm principle to maternal-fetal conflicts ethically justifiable? This question is complex and hard to answer for several reasons. The first relates to the moral standing of the fetus. The harm principle is intended to be applied to persons, to full members of the moral community. The question of whether a fetus at any stage in its development should be accorded the status of a person is unsettled and will no doubt remain so. But however that question might be resolved, the harm principle could still apply to a fetus who will become a person—the wanted fetus, of any gestational age. In this situation, a fetus can be said to have interests, not accruing to its current status as a fetus, but rather, to the infant and child it will later become. Thus, whether or not the fetus is a person is irrelevant to the application of the harm principle. What is relevant is that the wanted fetus will become a person, and so it has future-oriented interests.

The second reason why the applicability of the harm principle is problematic has to do with the degree of interference it licenses. How far is it permissible to go in forcing a woman to comply with an agreed upon standard of behavior during pregnancy? Efforts to persuade her, to cajole her, to convince her by reasoned argument and even by emotional appeals are all within acceptable bounds. These efforts may well be ineffective, especially since the behaviors in question are to a great degree physically or psychologically addictive. But should she be threatened with the sanctions of law, punished or incarcerated for failure to abstain from consuming alcohol, tobacco, and pharmaceutical as well as recreational drugs during pregnancy?

We believe she should not. Although a consequentialist analysis yields the judgment that a pregnant woman is under a moral obligation to abstain from behavior that risks the health or normal development of her fetus, no corresponding legal obligation should be put in place. Three different, but related considerations compel this conclusion.

First is the uncertainty surrounding risks to a particular fetus. Legally sanctioned interference with the freedom of pregnant women to consume what they wish would result in many more women being restricted than the number of fetuses that would actually be affected. With risks to the particular fetus remaining unclear, interfering with the behavior of all pregnant women would impose too harsh a restriction.

A second consideration builds on the first: incarceration even of those pregnant women whose fetuses would end up being harmed is the most restrictive alternative, and therefore, unacceptable. Few values in our society stand above those of individual liberty and autonomy. In other areas of the law, courts have mandated that the least restrictive measures be used to achieve desired ends. Although the birth of infants with abnormalities that could have been prevented is sad and may even be tragic, it is outweighed by the greater harm done by systematic interference with the freedom and autonomy of competent, adult women in our society.

The third consideration builds still further on the preceding ones. Additional unsavory consequences would flow from having legally sanctioned interference with the freedom of pregnant women. Knowing that they are at risk for incarceration or other punishment, pregnant women who persist in their health-risking behavior are likely to engage in patterns of lying and deception. How will laws and official policies be enforced? The prospect of invasions of privacy, in addition to interference with liberty, is another potential hazard. Who will police such laws? The woman's husband or other family members? Friends and neighbors? The most likely candidates are physicians and other health professionals.

Although it might be thought that ethical dilemmas pertaining to maternal-fetal conflict do not involve physicians and other health professionals, they cannot avoid playing some role. Even in the absence of laws that would require physicians delivering prenatal care to report instances of maternal drinking, smoking, or drug use, or to use surreptitious methods such as urine testing, physicians are likely to learn of the woman's habits. In a physician-patient relationship marked by cooperation and trust, the physician will ask the woman and she will probably respond truthfully about her behavior. What, then, is the obligation of physicians who become aware of this potentially harmful maternal behavior?

The physician has a duty to advise and counsel the woman about the risk her behavior poses both to herself and to her fetus. If, despite the counseling, the woman continues to engage in health-risking behavior, the physician has few choices. One possibility is to refuse to treat such a patient, but little is gained by this maneuver. Some physicians might decide to withdraw and insist that the woman find another physician, or assist her by recommending someone. The only other option is to attempt to optimize the treatment and continue the counseling, despite the patient's failure to comply with the physician's advice.

Finally, in addition to the negative effects of alcohol, drugs, and smoking in pregnancy, there are the potential negative effects of hazards in the workplace on the developing fetus. Few adequate studies have been done on the effects on the developing fetus of working with most chemicals and organic solvents. Recently, the National Institute for Occupational Safety and Health has reviewed the information currently available on chemical hazards in the workplace (32). In addition to concerns about the hazards of the chemical environment, there is increasing worry about the hazards of nonionizing radiation generated by microwave ovens, video display terminals, and other high-intensity sources of energy. There is also the known toxicity of anesthetic agents and other chemicals used in the medical setting. We have chosen not to address the public policy and political issues concerning hazards in the workplace, but rather to look at the maternal conflicts concerning her behavior.

Since approximately 43 percent of the civilian work force is now female and a large percentage of women are working not just for additional spending money but because the family has a basic need for that income, the consequentialist analysis of maternal obligations concerning behaviors during pregnancy is quite different when applied to hazards in the workplace than in the context of using alcohol, drugs, and tobacco.

If a woman is aware that the environment of her workplace may be potentially damaging to her developing fetus, is she obligated to seek alternative employment? The question becomes more complicated if it is unlikely that the woman will find an alternative job, in light of the large numbers of unemployed who are looking for positions. Furthermore, the alternative job might be at a salary substantially lower than her present position. The risk-benefit analysis in this ethical dilemma is thus rather complex. It includes not only the ambiguity of level of risk to the fetus, but the additional, quite different risk-benefit analysis of the trade-offs the woman faces for herself and her family.

There is little doubt that a hazard imposed on a developing fetus whose mother is determined to carry it to term can do as much long-term harm as a similar hazard imposed on a child after birth. In some circumstances, because the organs are in a critical developmental period, even more harm may be inflicted on an exposed fetus than on an exposed child. Thus the level of risk to the fetus may be assessed as substantial. Nevertheless, we believe that the consequentialist analysis must take all potential risks into account and not merely assume that the maternal and familial risks are unimportant.

The physician has little role in this potential area of conflict except to provide accurate information to the woman concerning the environmental risk of her occupation. It would be hard to imagine a physician feeling obligated to do more than clarify the facts and uncertainties of the situation in order for the woman to make an informed choice. Potential environmental hazards in the workplace seem to be increasing as we learn more about the various possible effects of chemicals and energy on the fetus. This will undoubtedly raise the level of concern and discourse in this area.

Conclusions

We have examined the ethical dilemmas created by the emerging area of fetal therapeutics and have suggested a framework for analysis of the potential conflicts. For experimental interventions, such as fetal surgery, we believe that women should be given all of the information necessary to make an informed choice and should not be coerced or obligated to consent to this research procedure. This conclusion is based on the very nature of research, in which outcomes are uncertain and participation is voluntary.

With regard to medical treatment of the woman in order to enhance fetal outcome, and maternal behaviors that pose risks to the developing fetus, we believe that the woman has a moral obligation to act in a manner that promotes the best interests of the fetus. However, we believe that the duty of the physician in these instances is limited to trying to convince the woman to comply with the recommended treatment or behavior; the physician's duty does not extend to initiating legal actions to attempt to ensure compliance. The physician may find it difficult to be sympathetic to the woman's refusal to act in the prescribed manner, and should use all available forms of moral persuasion to change the woman's mind, but should not be party to overriding the woman's autonomy by forcibly restraining or incarcerating her. This position is based on the principle of respect for persons, which gives rise to a duty to the woman that supersedes the duty to act beneficently to the fetus.

In the case of cesarean deliveries recommended for fetal indications, we believe that a consequentialist analysis yields the conclusion that a woman's refusal should be honored. A significantly increased risk of her dying during childbirth is sufficiently high to respect as binding her weighing of risks to herself from the surgery as greater than the potential risks to her fetus from foregoing the cesarean delivery. Although the medical risks and benefits can be objectively determined, a patient's assessment of the degree of risk she is willing to assume for the sake of predicted benefits is a subjective matter. Even when the degree of risk can be ascertained with some accuracy, based on well-documented statistics, reasonable people disagree on the question of which of life's risks are worth taking to attain desired benefits.

When it comes to established, efficacious treatments that pose low risk to the woman and great benefit to the fetus, such as blood transfusions given to the woman which are necessary to preserve the life or health of the fetus, we find ourselves in disagreement. One of us (A.R.F.) holds that it is acceptable for physicians to bring pressure to bear on the woman to accept the procedure, including the coercive step of seeking court adjudication. However, coercive measures should stop short of physically restraining or forcibly sedating a woman who continues to refuse treatment despite a court order that grants physicians permission to override her refusal. The other of us (R.M.) would allow persuasive efforts, emotional appeals, and other noncoercive means to convince a woman to accept a low-risk medical procedure for the sake of her fetus, but holds it unacceptable to invoke the force of law to override her refusal.

There is a natural tendency to describe this situation as one of overwhelming benefits to the fetus, which, when balanced against the minor risks to the pregnant woman, justify the suspension of her right to refuse medical treatment. According to this analysis, the woman's right should be honored unless the risks to her are so minimal and the benefits to the fetus so great as to warrant overriding that right. Our disagreement would then rest on the problem of line drawing. When are the risks to the woman sufficiently great to allow her to maintain her autonomy, and when are the benefits to her fetus sufficiently great to justify overriding her autonomy? The problem with an analysis along these lines is that it mixes the two ethical frameworks we have argued should be kept separate.

Another possible mode of analysis adheres consistently to a consequentialist framework, but holds that the determination of risks and benefits is a subjective matter, one that depends on each individual's values and personal preferences. The explanation of our disagreement would then rest on a difference in our respective assignments of the degree of risks and benefits. This, too, is an unacceptable way of characterizing our disagreement, since we maintain that the assignment of risks and benefits is based on objectively determined scientific data. If the assessment of risks and benefits were entirely subjective, there would be no basis for a physician's claim to expertise in these matters over that of the woman, and hence, no basis for seeking a court order on the grounds that the risks to the woman are minimal while the benefits to the fetus are great. However, as we have noted, the weight a person assigns to these objectively determined risks and benefits, the way they are used in coming to a decision, is a subjective matter, depending, among other things, on whether one is inclined to take risks or tends to be risk-averse.

The best explanation for our disagreement on this issue is one that retains the consequentialist framework, yet at the same time shows that using that framework is no simple matter. The one of us who would seek a court order to permit physicians to override the woman's refusal of blood transfusions and other low-risk procedures is a physician, whose primary role in the medical setting is to bring about the best outcomes for his patients. In the typical situation of weighing risks and benefits to a single patient, the physician uses objectively determined risks and benefits and recommends treatment based on a favorable benefit-risk ratio. In the two-patient situation, the calculation is somewhat more complex but proceeds along the same lines. The risks and benefits to each patient must be assessed, and the treatment recommendation based on a favorable overall balance of benefits over risks. This application of the consequentialist framework draws boundaries around the specific patients to whom the physician is obligated—the woman and her fetus in the particular medical situation. Considering the benefits and risks to both patients, the physician judges that the best consequences, on the whole, lie in seeking a court order to undertake the procedures.

How narrowly or broadly the consequences of actions should be construed is itself a value-laden decision. This is the basis for our disagreement. The bioethicist does not have professional role obligations to particular patients and can thus cast the consequentialist net more widely than the physician. The one of us who would not seek a court order performs a calculation that includes consequences for other patients and for the society as a whole. A society in which physicians invoke the force of law against women for the sake of their infants-to-be, and in which patients (women in this case) are held hostage to the health or normalcy of the children they will bear is less desirable than a society that respects the autonomy of competent, adult patients even in circumstances where their refusal of treatment can result in a poor outcome for a fetus, soon to become an infant.

Thus, while adhering to the consequentialist framework for conducting an ethical analysis, we differ in how we would apply that framework. The conclusion that one of us (A.R.F.) reaches stems from the role obligations of the physician: to bring about the best consequences for the patient—in this case, the two patients. The consequentialist analysis does not require the impossible balancing of the rights of fetus and pregnant woman, and it avoids the problems of ascribing rights to the fetus. It gives equal consideration to both patients, coming down on the side of seeking a court order for a procedure that presents a low risk to the woman and considerable benefit to the fetus. The conclusion that the other of us (R.M.) reaches stems from a broader consideration of the consequences, extending beyond the particular patients in a given case to future patients and the larger societal implications of condoning coercion by physicians and involving legal mechanisms in an ongoing way in the medical setting.

These divergent conclusions, both using a consequentialist framework, do not reveal an inherent flaw in consequentialism. The different conclusions we arrive at reflect an underlying debate in philosophical ethics between two versions of utilitarianism: act utilitarianism and rule utilitarianism. The first requires an assessment of the consequences of each individual act, mandating the action that produces the best consequences for the affected parties. The second assesses the consequences of having a general practice or policy, comprising many individual actions, and judges the rightness or wrongness of individual acts by whether they comport with the general practice determined to have the best overall consequences. Neither of these versions of utilitarianism is obviously right or wrong. Even among those who find a consequentialist analysis superior to a rights-based analysis, disagreement persists concerning whether act utilitarianism or rule utilitarianism is to be preferred when they yield different conclusions. Understanding these differences and the sources of disagreement are important for being able to resolve controversial issues in a rational and enlightened manner.

Enhanced knowledge concerning fetal assessment, fetal therapy, and the risks to the fetus posed by the environment has created some new areas of interest to biomedical ethics. Because of the unique relationship between the pregnant woman and her fetus, physically, emotionally, and morally, the ethical analysis of potential conflicts between these two actors is quite complex. A careful consequentialist analysis, assessing potential risks and benefits, has the greatest prospect for clarifying this new and exciting field, and helping to resolve the dilemmas that are bound to arise.

References

1. Harrison MR. Unborn: historical perspective of the fetus as a patient. Pharos 1982;45:19–24.
2. Lenow JL. The fetus as a patient: emerging rights as a person. Am J Law Med 1983;9:1–29.
3. Fletcher JC. The fetus as patient: ethical issues. JAMA 1981;246:772–73.
4. Bowes WA, Selgestad B. Fetal versus maternal rights: Medical and legal perspectives. Obstet Gynecol 1981;58:209–14.
5. Ruddick W, Wilcox W. Operating on the fetus. Hastings Cent Rep 1982;12:10–14.
6. National Commission for the Protection of Human Subjects. The Belmont report. Washington DC: US Government Printing Office, 1979.
7. Chervenak FA, McCullough LB. Perinatal ethics: a practical method of analysis of obligation to mother and fetus. Obstet Gynecol 1985;66:442–46.
8. Merkatz IR, Adam PAJ, eds. The diabetic pregnancy: a perinatal perspective. New York: Grune and Stratton, 1979.
9. Robertson JA. Legal issues in fetal therapy. Semin Perinatol 1985;9:136–142.
10. Collaborative Group on Antenatal Steroid Therapy. Effect of antenatal dexamethasone administration on the prevention of respiratory distress syndrome. Am J Obstet Gynecol 1981;141:276–86.

11. Schulman JD. Prenatal treatment of biochemical disorders. Semin Perinatol 1985;9:75–78.
12. Ampola MG, Mahoney MJ, Nakamura E, et al. Prenatal therapy of a patient with vitamin responsive methylmalonic acidemia. N Engl J Med 1975;293:313–15.
13. Kleinman CS, Donnerstein RL, Jaffe CC, et al. Fetal echocardiography—a tool for evaluation of in utero cardiac arrhythmias and monitoring of in utero therapy. Am J Cardiol 1983;51:237–43.
14. Liley AW. Intrauterine transfusion of foetus in haemolytic disease. Br Med M 1963;2:1107–9.
15. Peddle LJ. The antenatal management of the Rh sensitized woman. Clin Perinatol 1984;11:251–66.
16. Clewell WH, Meier PR, Manchester DK, et al. Ventriculomegaly: evaluation and management. Semin Perinatol 1985;9:98–102.
17. Golbus MS, Filly RA, Callen PW, et al. Fetal urinary tract obstruction: management and selection for treatment. Semin Perinatol 1985;9:91–97.
18. Harrison MR, Adzick NS, Nakayama DK, deLorimier AA. Fetal diaphragmatic hernia: fatal but fixable. Semin Perinatol 1985;9:103–112.
19. Harrison MR, Filly RA, Golbus MS, et al. Fetal treatment 1982. N Engl J Med 1982;307:1651–52.
20. 45 CFR 46, Federal Register 46, No 16, Jan 26, 1981, p 8366–91.
21. Annas GJ. Forced cesareans: the most unkindest cut of all. Hastings Cent Rep 1982;12:16–17.
22. Fletcher JC. Emerging ethical issues in fetal therapy. In: Research ethics. New York: Alan R Liss, pp 293–318.
23. Fleischman AR. The immediate impact of the birth of a low birth weight infant on the family. Zero to three 1986;4:1–5.
24. Macklin R. Fetal therapy: new ethical issues or old? In: Humber JM, Almeder RT, eds., Biomedical ethics reviews. Clifton NJ: Humana Press, 1984.
25. Hubbard R. The fetus as patient. Ms, Oct 1982, p 32.
26. Macklin R. Moral concerns and appeals to rights and duties. Hastings Cent Rep 1976;6:31–38.
27. Clewell WH, Johnson ML, Meier PR, et al. A surgical approach to the treatment of fetal hydrocephalus. N Engl J Med 1982;306:1320–25.
28. Fleischman AR, Murray T. Ethics committees for Infants Doe? An alternative that deserves a chance. Hastings Cent Rep 1983;13:5–9.
29. Bross IDJ, Natarajan N. Genetic damage from diagnostic radiation. JAMA 1977;237:2399–2401.
30. Jones KL, Smith DW, Ulleland CN, et al. Patterns of malformation in offspring of chronic alcoholic women. Lancet 1973;1:1267.
31. Jones KL, Chernoff GF. Effects of chemical and environmental agents on fetal development in maternal-fetal medicine. In: Creasy RK, Resnick R, eds., Maternal-Fetal Medicine. Philadelphia: WB Saunders, 1984, pp 189–200.
32. National Institute for Occupational Safety and Health. Current intelligence bulletin. Morbidity Mortality Weekly Rep 1985;34:33S–51S.

IV

Postnatal Period

6

Quality of Life in Neonatal Ethics: Beyond Denial and Evasion

JOHN D. ARRAS

Should the anticipated quality of a child's life matter to those charged with making life-or-death decisions in the neonatal nursery? Is it ethical for caregivers and parents to weigh a child's physical disabilities or mental impairments in deciding whether or not to deploy life-sustaining medical treatments? All parties to the debate over the proper care of seriously anomalous or disabled neonates concur that this is the fundamental question. Unfortunately, this is where their agreement ends. The so-called pro-life faction strenuously denies the moral legitimacy of all quality-of-life judgments as applied to the care of imperiled newborns (1), whereas the other side affirms the appropriateness, and indeed the inevitability, of quality-of-life reasoning (2).

Notwithstanding its pivotal role in the debate over seriously impaired newborns, the concept of "quality of life" has remained largely unanalyzed and poorly understood. The advocates of quality-of-life reasoning rarely pause to argue why the quality of a person's life should count or to specify in detail exactly what qualitative conditions ought to ground moral argument. The abstractness and vagueness of most quality-of-life arguments have led many to suspect that invocations of quality of life merely function to mask the assertion of unbridled subjectivity and selfishness on the part of caregivers and parents. Although the proponents of quality of life have often fallen far short of making a persuasive case, the complete debasement of this concept has fallen to the opposition. In the hands of pro-life partisans, "quality of life" has come to assume the status of a code word for a willingness to kill any child that is less than perfect. Although the term was no doubt originally coined by persons motivated by compassion for the victims of an unrelenting and often unfeeling application of high-technology medicine, pro-life advocates have largely succeeded in their efforts to impute the

The author would like to thank Nancy Dubler, Liz Emrey, Alan Fleischman, Nancy Rhoden, Stephen Wear, and Connie Zuckerman for many helpful comments on a draft of this chapter.

motives of selfishness and disregard for the handicapped to anyone who would factor quality of life into moral decision making. Objectionable connotations are now so intimately fused in public discourse with the very concept of quality of life that even its proponents no longer dare speak its name. It is indeed a sad commentary on this public debate to note that innuendo and euphemism have all too often taken the place of honest disagreement and straightforward argument.

The purpose of this chapter is to retrieve the concept of quality of life from this miasma of misunderstanding, suspicion, and evasion. My aims are twofold: first, to clarify the concept of quality of life; and second, to argue for an ethic based on a suitably hedged understanding of quality of life. I first sketch the emergence of this concept against the background of technological innovation in medicine. I then argue that in spite of many legitimate (and some spurious) reservations concerning the quality of life, resort to this concept is not only morally appropriate, but actually unavoidable. Finally, I undertake an extensive analysis of the term "quality of life," focusing on such questions as: Whose quality of life should be considered? From which point of view should the quality of the infant's life be determined? And what is the lower limit of "acceptable" quality of life?

Instead of undertaking a comprehensive analysis of the ethics of newborn care, I have attempted to limit the scope of this essay in two ways. First, in cleaving to my assigned topic, the quality of life, I have had to bracket a number of important questions that would have to figure prominently in any truly comprehensive treatment of the subject. (For example, the question of who should decide—parents, caregivers, the government? And what should be the scope of their legitimate discretion?) Second, this essay does not even pretend to be an exhaustive gloss on the quality-of-life problem. I have, for example, omitted entirely the crucial issue of whether a *morally* acceptable standard of quality of life ought to be relegated entirely to the sphere of private decision making, or whether it should rather be *publicly* articulated, publicly validated, and openly inscribed in our legal rules and social policies. Due to the possibly adverse social consequences of publicly establishing a quality-of-life threshold, some observers have stressed the difference between privately *using* quality-of-life reasoning in certain cases and *saying* publicly that we use it (3). This issue, to which I shall return in a subsequent essay, is too important to tack onto an already lengthy chapter.

Quality of Life and the Technological Imperative

The Emergence of 'Quality of Life'

Prior to the advent of scientific medicine and high-technology mechanisms for preserving life, there was probably not much use for the concept "quality of life." Apart from bleeding, blistering, and purging—themselves treatments of dubious efficacy—medicine could not do very much to cure illness and prolong life (4). (Indeed, most standard aggressive treatments probably did more harm than good.) Those who were seriously ill either recovered spontaneously or got worse and died. To insist on quality of life in an era when physicians could do little to prolong life would have made little sense.

Once physicians began to understand the nature and mechanisms of disease, however, it became possible not merely to diagnose, but to intervene. Lives could be saved and improved through the intercession of scientifically developed therapeutics. More important, the development of the modern intensive care unit—with its respirators, monitors, vasopressors, and other "miracles"—signaled our emerging ability to stay the hand of death, not only from patients suffering acute but reversible illnesses, but also from the moribund and the "hopeless" (5). Soon the dark side of modern medicine began to take on definable form: physicians trained to "save lives" through the aggressive application of medical technology were beginning to achieve rather questionable results. Otherwise competent individuals found that, once they had stepped on the escalator of high-technology medicine, they could not get off. They were, quite literally, "prisoners of the ICU" (6). Moreover, it soon became apparent that, for many patients, the mere prolongation of life was not an ultimate and absolute value, especially when the life prolonged was marked by little more than pain, suffering, and indignity. The quality of a person's life, as opposed to its sheer quantitative extension, had finally become an issue.

"Quality of life" as a concept in moral argument thus derived from a perceived need to "humanize" the practice of contemporary medicine (7). A way had to be found to discriminate between the indisputably beneficial uses of the new technology and those which merely seemed to heap new, unanticipated burdens onto the human condition. The notion of quality of life originally functioned, then, as a salutary check on the unthinking and often unfeeling deployment of life-preserving medical technologies in situations where they did little good and much harm to patients and their families.

In stark contrast to the connotation of quality of life in pro-life circles today, the values animating the emergence of this concept were unobjectionable, even noble. To insist on a concern for the quality of life was to insist on the importance of individual freedom, dignity, and mercy in the face of an implacable technological imperative. Prolonged dying in the hospital with tubes protruding from every conceivable orifice, with every failing function monitored to perfection, an intern pounding on your chest in the final ebbing moments, was rightly added to the modern catalogue of horrors.

Quality of Life in the Debate Over Newborns

Moving from the emergence of the term "quality of life" in the 1950s and 1960s to its role in today's Baby Doe debate, we will have to be much more specific about the meaning and functions of the concept in this new context. Lofty and abstract invocations of human freedom and dignity in the face of unrelenting technology retain their resonance, to be sure, but they fail to define the issues with adequate precision. What does it mean to argue for quality of life in the neonatal intensive care unit?

We should begin by asking, Quality of life *as opposed to what?* What alternatives are there to an ethic of caring for newborns based on a concern for the quality of their lives? One alternative, which I shall call "vitalism," holds that, so long as the patient lives, every reasonable effort must be made to prolong the patient's life. Mere biological existence, in other words, constitutes a compelling reason to continue aggressive treatments (8). From this rather extreme perspective, it matters not whether the life that is being preserved is of high or low quality to its possessor—or indeed whether or not the patient is even conscious of having a life. All that matters is the brute fact of human life. Where there is life, even life that has entered the process of its own dying, there exists a strict duty to perpetuate it.

So defined, "vitalism" suffers from two major difficulties. First, the strict moral duty to preserve valiantly all human life, no matter how moribund and bereft of value even to its possessor, lacks a coherent and plausible moral justification. Given the crushing moral and economic costs of such an ethic, more than mere moral intuition will have to be offered to justify the claim that human existence per se, quite apart from its value or quality, calls for the continuous application of medical technology. Second, and perhaps even more devastating, this extremist version of vitalism has virtually no defenders. Even the most vociferous critics of quality of life reasoning—from theologians like Paul Ramsey (9) to C. Everett Koop, surgeon general and point man in President Reagan's campaign on behalf of handicapped infants (10)—willingly admit that there is no ethical or legal imperative to prolong the lives of dying patients. This sort of vitalism, then, is actually more an abstract and empty placemarker for the most extreme position imaginable than a viable ethical option in the Baby Doe debate.

The real theoretical alternative to a quality-of-life position in neonatal ethics, the position that will give our concept its required specificity in this context, is what Ramsey has called a "medical indications" policy (9). According to this view, medical treatments may not be morally withheld from infants except 1) when the infant has entered into the process of his or her own dying, or 2) when the physician concludes using "reasonable medical judgment" that a particular intervention will not "help" or offer a "net benefit" to the infant. Thus, if a child is perceived to be in the process of dying (whatever that is), caregivers need not press the use of further curative measures. For example, if suffering from catastrophic intracranial hemorrhage and multiple system failures that together signal imminent death, a child need not have her death prolonged by resort to kidney dialysis and heavy-duty vasopressors.

Likewise, if a physician believes that a proposed therapeutic intervention will not work or be truly effective, there is no moral obligation to try. If, for example, a newborn presents with a life-threatening cardiac lesion but his physicians believe that operating immediately would pose even greater risks to his life, then surgery is not medically or morally "indicated." (Although this sort of example is clear enough, we shall see later that the question of which treatments are "truly effective" or "beneficial" for a particular infant is a matter of important controversy.)

Whereas the medical indications policy thus allows two exceptions to the moral imperative to treat anomalous or impaired infants, that is all it allows. Significantly, it disallows any and all nontreatment decisions based on estimates of the child's future mental or physical disabilities— that is, on the child's quality of life. So long as a child is not engaged in the process of dying, and so long as physicians believe that a proposed treatment is medically indicated, then that treatment must be given. Reasons relating to the child's future quality of life—for example, that he will never walk, hold a job, marry, recognize his caretakers, be free from constant and intractable pain—are ruled out as being strictly *irrelevant* from a moral point of view.

We are finally ready to give a positive account of what would constitute a quality-of-life ethic in the context of the debate over imperiled newborns. Any such ethic will assert that, in addition to the exceptions already elaborated by the medical indications policy, caregivers may morally withhold life-sustaining care from *nondying* infants on grounds relating to the quality of the patient's present and future life (11). According to such a theory, the fact that a child's life will be marked (for example) by pain, suffering, and isolation is a morally relevant aspect of the situation and could therefore provide a reason for discontinuing treatment and allowing the child to die. As will be shown later, however, this minimal definition of a quality-of-life position is sufficiently broad to shelter a wide variety of distinct (and in some cases, incompatible) ethical theories and conclusions regarding the care of imperiled newborns. No progress can be made on the ultimate question—namely, Should quality of life matter?—until we have specified *which* quality-of-life theory we wish to scrutinize.

Objections and Reservations

In spite of its noble lineage in our struggle to temper the use of medical technologies, and in spite of its initial plausibility in the neonatal context, the notion of quality of life has been attacked, dismissed, or disowned by just about every major participant in recent Baby Doe debates. What are the major arguments against allowing *any* quality-of-life considerations in neonatal treatment decisions?

Impossibility

The first argument is based on two special features of quality-of-life judgments in this particular context. First, such judgments will always be made on behalf of the infant by some other party, usually the parents in conjunction with the child's physicians. Although skeptics might be perfectly comfortable with first-person quality-of-life judgments, in which competent adults base their own treatment decisions on personal values and their own estimates of their future quality of life, they balk at our ability to make such judgments for others. Second, the particular kind of quality-of-life judgment called for in the Baby Doe debate would have us compare, not merely better life against worse life for the same individual, but life as it is versus no life at all. With the sole exception of theories that sanction nontreatment for the good of others, all quality-of-life approaches implicitly or explicitly affirm the proposition that in certain circumstances infants are better off dead than alive.

The first argument concludes from these two observations that the particular kind of quality-of-life judgment called for here is impossible to make (9). It is one thing to choose life with quality X over life with quality Y; it is another to choose death over life of any particular sort. The latter judgment, it is alleged, founders on conceptual incoherence. Just as "killing for peace" involves its defenders in self-contradiction, so too does the notion of someone's being "better off dead." As Ramsey puts it, "No one can weigh life against nothingness. . . . [N]o one can look into the chasm between life and death and weigh the difference— not without first being alive, which makes quite a difference"(9: pp. 206–7).

Whatever we might want to say about this argument, we should note that it quickly involves its advocates in their own self-contradiction. While it is obviously true that one must first be alive in order to compare the respective merits of life and death, this fact does nothing to under- mine the intelligibility of choosing to end one's life sooner rather than later. Indeed, Ramsey and the other theorists who have popularized this argument see nothing incoherent, or even necessarily wrong, in a com- petent adult choosing an earlier death on grounds of an unacceptable quality of life (9: pp. 154–59). If so, they must concede that, for such individuals, it makes sense to choose an early death in favor of an excessively burdensome future. But this stance involves us in the very comparison of existence with nonexistence that Ramsey says is "essen- tially incoherent." Thus, Ramsey assumes the intelligibility of such judgments when made by competent adults in the course of exercising their right to refuse life-sustaining treatments, but he denies their coher- ence when made on behalf of impaired newborns. Since we are arguing intelligibility and logical coherence rather than wisdom or morality here, Ramsey cannot have it both ways. Either comparisons of life with non- life are possible or they are not. Whatever a clever philosopher might say by way of a constructive defense of such comparisons, we need merely note here that if such judgments are not logically coherent, then the moribund cancer patient who refuses a final round of painful chemo- therapy, the captured spy who kills herself rather than reveal secrets, and all others who knowingly shorten their lives rather than live a certain kind of life—then all such persons have a good deal of explaining to do. Do we really want to say that all such actions are based on a principle that is irrational and incoherent?

Impropriety

The fallback position for critics of quality-of-life judgments is to assert that, while such judgments may not be impossible, they are at least morally wrong on principle. Even if it makes logical sense for one person to choose death for another (in this case, for an imperiled newborn), that person, so the argument goes, has no *right* to do so. We may well have the right to refuse life-sustaining treatments for ourselves (in other words to choose an earlier death) but, it is said, we have no right to make this kind of life-and-death choice for other persons. Only *they* have the moral right to pass final judgment on the quality of their own lives. Only they can know what is the limit of acceptable life for them.

This is a more plausible argument. It is based on the existence of tremendous variability between people on questions of value (the meaning of life) and on our differing capacities to endure pain and suffering. Whereas some people steadfastly refuse to "go gentle into that good night," no matter how intense their suffering, others (like myself) have a rather limited capacity for unremitting physical pain and psychological suffering. On such fundamental and personal matters as the meaning of life and the limits of suffering, no one has the right, it is said, to answer for another.

This argument is strongest in those situations where we can expect significant variability in response to the question, "Is this life worth living?" There is definitely something morally suspect, for example, about a highly intellectual couple choosing death for their mildly retarded child on the ground that "Nobody could possibly want to live like that." Here we are likely to say that this couple indeed have no right to impose their fastidious standards of mental functioning on their child.

But suppose that instead of mild retardation, their child suffers unremitting and intractable pain due to some medical condition; and that even if he is treated aggressively, he will die from another incurable anomaly before his first birthday. Would we still maintain, in this second situation, that the parents have no right to withhold life-sustaining treatments from their grievously afflicted child? I think not, and rightly so.

Ordinarily, when we say that someone has no right to choose for another, we are likely to assume that if the latter could speak for himself, he might well choose differently. But what if treatment is withheld, as in this example, not for selfish or idiosyncratic reasons, but for reasons that most unbiased onlookers would regard as beyond reproach: for example, mercifully sparing their child from a very short life of horrible suffering? In this event, I think it would be quite odd for someone to say, "Yes, the parents acted mercifully in withdrawing painful treatment from their tragically afflicted child, and on balance it was probably the best thing they could have done for her; yet they had no right to do so." To insist on each person's right to make his own choices regarding the meaning of life and the limits of suffering in such catastrophic cases would, I submit, be tantamount to making a fetish out of autonomy and a prison house out of the notion of rights. It would be to reduce a morally complex situation—in which a legitimate regard for mercy ought to co-exist with respect for the individual (future) wishes of the patient—to an overly simple (indeed, simplistic) ethic of autonomy. When we can no longer ask, "What is the *good* for this child?" (a child, by the way, who will *ex hypothesi* never be able to express his preferences to us), when we have reached the point where a single-minded concern for the "rights" of the child eclipses all other concerns, including a legitimate and merciful concern for the physical and psychological well-being of the child, then at this point the notion of rights assumes a frightening autonomy and turns against the human good. Parents who act selfishly or wrongly with regard to their own impaired children, parents who contravene the good of their children, indeed have no right to do so. But if parents act so as to advance the good of their children, even if this means withholding life-sustaining treatments and permitting an early death, then they certainly have a right to do so. If they do not, who else does? If no one does, who will be left to act for the good of the child?

Clearly, then, the issue of whether parents have the right to make life-and-death decisions for their children is subordinate to the more basic question of whether the parents are advancing the good of their child. Of course, the nature of this good can be exceedingly difficult to ascertain in particular circumstances, but that is no reason to allow a hypertrophic concept of individual rights to preclude this painful but necessary inquiry.

Prognostic Uncertainty

Even if we grant the basic presupposition of most quality-of-life theories—namely, that some conditions can be so horrible that death is a good, or at least a lesser evil, to the afflicted person—we often face formidable problems in attempting to predict which infants will suffer those conditions. Even if we can achieve *moral* agreement on the proper criteria of nontreatment, we may lack an adequate *factual* base on which to ground our moral judgments. Prognostication in the delivery room or the neonatal nursery is a notoriously risky business. In many, if not most, cases physicians cannot predict with a reasonable degree of certitude whether or to what extent a child will suffer from impairments in later life (12). A Down syndrome child or a baby with a grade 4 intracranial bleed may or may not turn out to be profoundly retarded. Many do, but many do not. In the face of such prognostic uncertainty, how can we opt for death when, for all the doctors know, a particular child might, if given the chance, turn out to have a life well worth living?

Interpreted as a cautionary reminder of our human fallibility, this argument must be taken seriously. When the issue is life versus death, and when our actions or omissions will yield irreversible consequences, prudence and caution are certainly the best policy. Life-sustaining treatment should not be withheld from an infant unless her physicians can state, with a reasonable degree of medical certitude, that the child's impairments will render her life disproportionately burdensome. If physicians cannot offer such reasonable assurances, then the decision makers should probably err on the side of preserving life.

Interpreted as a definitive refutation of all quality-of-life positions, however, this argument surely goes too far. This is because there are some conditions that can be diagnosed with exactitude and whose sequelae are eminently predictable. Trisomy 13, trisomy 18, and cri-du-chat and several other syndromes are known to involve severe mental retardation and a host of extremely serious cardiac, gastrointestinal, and growth-related abnormalities (13). (The two trisomies are also invariably linked to a very short life span—one to two years, at most.) In addition, other conditions that cannot be diagnosed with the exactitude of the chromosomal abnormalities above can be assessed with some degree of reasonable medical certainty. Take, for example, a child born with massive hydrocephalus (55 cm in circumference, say, as opposed to the normal 35 cm), gross brain abnormalities and malformations (including destroyed vision centers in the brain), and an unusually large and high spina bifida lesion. I take it that, in such a case, physicians can reasonably predict that the child will be blind, severely retarded, permanently paralyzed, incontinent of both urine and feces, permanently crib-bound, and most likely never able to recognize his caretakers. In order to live this particular life, the child will have to undergo painful skin grafting, numerous shuntings, and scores of major and minor surgical interventions. Supposing that we can reach sufficient *moral* certainty in determining that such a life is so burdensome as to justify nontreatment? I would contend that the degree of *medical* certainty achievable in such cases is sufficient for the admittedly quite grave purposes of our inquiry.

Subjectivity

The final objection we shall consider to the very concept of quality-of-life reasoning builds on yet another feature of most quality-of-life positions: their vagueness. Quality of life can mean a wide variety of things to different people. To some it may mean an overweaning concern for normalcy; any deviations from the norm will not be tolerated. To others it may mean a willingness to tolerate all but the most catastrophic forms of anomaly and impairment. Between these extremes, still others fill in an entire spectrum of standards of "acceptable life" on the basis of their own experiences, values, capacities, and needs.

Given the vagueness of most statements about it, critics argue, the phrase "quality of life" tends to give free reign to the *subjective preferences* of decision makers (14). For example, the American Medical Association, in response to the Reagan administration's Baby Doe rule, has stated that "[q]uality of life is a factor to be considered in determining what is best for the individual. Life should be cherished despite disabilities and handicaps, except when prolongation would be inhumane and unconscionable" (15). The problem, of course, is how to define what constitutes "inhumane and unconscionable" conditions of human life. Presumably, different people will define these terms in different ways, with varying degrees of strictness. It is argued that the vagueness of such a standard would allow decision makers to do whatever they wanted, provided they were willing to justify the result as an alternative to an inhumane and unconscionable prolongation of life. To make allowances for quality-of-life reasoning would thus clear the way for the free play of subjectivity, and would end in widespread abuse and neglect.

This argument is somewhat difficult to interpret due to the elusiveness of its concept of "subjectivity." What do the partisans of this objection mean by the term? They could mean that quality-of-life reasoning requires the application of individual human judgment, which is subjective in the sense that individuals must engage in a process of reasoning and come to some kind of conclusion on their own. But if this is what they mean, then the objection would abolish all ethical discretion, all scope for personal judgment in practical ethics. It would enthrone what philosopher Stephen Toulmin has called the "tyranny of principles" and signal an inhuman, inflexible retreat from the ethical realities of concrete situations (16).

Alternatively, they could mean by "subjective" reasons that have more to do with selfish or idiosyncratic desires of people than with what is called for by correct moral principles. But if this is the case, the solution would seem to be, not the abolition of all quality-of-life reasoning, but rather much greater care in the articulation and rational justification of principles based on quality-of-life reasoning. In addition to this kind of theoretical hedge against "subjectivity," we could also erect certain *procedural safeguards,* such as hospital ethics committees (17), against the subjective inclinations of those who would misinterpret or misapply the correct moral principles for their own purposes. Perhaps this dual strategy is as close as we can get to any meaningful notion of "objectivity" in this context.

The Inevitability of Quality-of-Life Judgments

So far, I have tried to show that the usual objections to the very idea of quality-of-life arguments are either untenable (for example, "Quality-of-life judgments are essentially incoherent," "We have no right to make them") or that they err by attempting to stretch good reasons for caution and prudence (the problems of prognostication and vagueness) into arguments against all quality-of-life arguments as such. Having shown that quality-of-life determinations are at least conceptually coherent and possibly morally permissible, I now want to demonstrate that, unless we are willing to embrace vitalism, we must accept quality-of-life judgments as an *inevitable* feature of any acceptable neonatal ethic. My strategy will be to review a variety of positions that either expressly disavow reasoning about "quality of life" or studiously avoid mention of the words. I shall examine the views of theological and secular ethicists, and the positions of various courts and governmental agencies. In each case, I will show how quality-of-life judgments play an essential role in the thinking of those who officially disavow them.

Weber's Theological Rejection

Although this is clearly not the place for a synoptic overview of contemporary theological ethics on the question of Baby Doe, the views of theologian Leonard Weber are typical and particularly instructive for our purposes (18, 19). Weber begins by opposing a "sanctity of life" ethic to a quality-of-life ethic, rejecting the latter on the ground that it "risk[s] the danger of saying that one person is more valuable than another because of his condition." He warns of the need for "protection against an arbitrary decision being made on the basis of a judgment about the worth of a particular type of life."

Interestingly, when Weber develops his own positive theoretical framework for approaching the Baby Doe controversy, he adopts the traditional distinction between "ordinary and extraordinary" means. According to this traditional view, treatments may be ethically forgone if they do not promise "reasonable hope of success" or if they threaten to impose "excessive burdens." In the latter category, Weber includes further treatments on severely brain damaged patients. Weber writes, "One can even talk about treatment imposing an excessive burden when it is the timing of the treatment that results in a *burdensome life* [my italics]. . . . By saving the life of the [extensively brain damaged] patient *at this time*, an excessive burden would be imposed. [Richard] Mc-Cormick and others would probably say that the decision not to treat in such a case is based on concern for the quality of the life of the child. And, of course, they are largely correct."

Weber thus draws my own conclusion for me: the traditional theological-ethical distinction between "ordinary and extraordinary" means, correctly interpreted, necessarily involves quality-of-life assessments. Simply put, in order to know whether a proposed treatment is "*excessively* burdensome," we have to know what kind of life that treatment will make possible. If it will merely be marked by pain and suffering, or by profound brain damage, then a good case could be made that the treatment is "extraordinary" (can be ethically foregone).

Weber's real objection, then, turns out not to be against quality-of-life *judgments*, which he admits are morally acceptable, but rather against quality-of-life *language*. The language of "extraordinary means" is preferable, according to Weber, because (he thinks that) its emphasis on the treatment itself will provide vulnerable patients with an extra measure of protection against arbitrary judgments based on the low quality of the patient's life. This is an important and interesting objection, but it is entirely unrelated to the question of whether we can actually do without quality-of-life judgments in this area. For his part, theologian Weber appears to admit that we cannot.

Secular 'Best Interests' Standards

Several important writers (20–22) and the influential President's Commission on bioethics (23) have recently fashioned a moderate third way between the extremes of a rigid "sanctity of life" (or "medical indications") policy and a highly permissive ethic that regards newborns as interchangeable "nonpersons." While concluding that not all nondying newborns need be kept alive, these writers and the President's Commission have insisted that the impaired child's effect on the well-being of others should be regarded as morally irrelevant to deliberations in the neonatal nursery and that our sole focus of attention should be the "best interests of the child." The moral attractiveness of this standard derives, in large part, from its very moderation: it sanctions some selective nontreatment decisions, but it does so from morally high ground by refusing to submerge the infant's life and worth in dubious interpersonal estimations of "social worth."

The best interests of the child standard is obviously premised on quality-of-life considerations. Speaking of nondying but severely impaired children, the President's Commission states that "permanent handicaps justify a decision not to provide life-sustaining treatment only when they are so severe that continued existence would not be a net benefit to the infant" (23). In other words, certain tragic impairments can make the lives of some children so miserable that they would be better off dead. Likewise, commentator Robert F. Weir embraces a "best interests" standard on the basis of the "principle of nonmaleficence" (that is, "above all, do no harm") (20: p. 199). He argues cogently that although death is in most circumstances viewed as an evil to be avoided, it is not always the ultimate form of harm. Indeed, in certain cases the pain and suffering attendant upon certain conditions combines with the iatrogenic toll of ineffective therapies to make continued existence a fate worse than death (20: pp. 199–208).

Although both the President's Commission and Weir explicitly reject a strict medical indications policy and obviously employ quality-of-life reasoning in erecting their best-interests standard, neither explicitly acknowledges the propriety, let alone the inevitability, of quality-of-life judgments. Weir canvasses a number of theories explicitly based on quality-of-life projections (among them the theories of Richard McCormick, Joseph Fletcher, and Jonathan Glover) but then moves on to articulate and embrace his own preferred best-interests standard as a distinct alternative to a quality-of-life position (20: pp. 164–70). Weir's reason for distancing himself from an explicit quality-of-life position—namely, that some of the partisans of quality of life permit interpersonal comparisons and trade-offs between the infant's good and that of others—does not explain why a separate category was needed, rather than a further refinement of the quality-of-life position.

The President's Commission's chapter on "Seriously Ill Newborns" (23) does not even mention the child's quality of life as a factor to be taken into account. (In fact, "quality of life" does not even appear in the index of the Commission's volume titled *Deciding to Forego Life-Sustaining Treatment*.) Throughout this chapter, references to the child's "best interests" and "well-being" consistently function as substitutes for the child's quality of life.

Why did the President's Commission studiously avoid referring to the concept of quality of life? My hunch is that the Commission's highest priority, here as in its other reports, was the achievement of a broad-based consensus (24). Realizing that their powers were purely advisory and that the problem they confronted was the subject of a heated and divisive public debate, the commissioners must have avoided all references to quality of life in order to avoid controversy and achieve consensus. Since the notion of quality of life had already achieved the status of a code word for the slaughter of the innocents, and since the commissioners had found a way to drape quality-of-life conclusions in the more acceptable language of the child's "best interests," dropping the offending phrase no doubt made a good deal of political sense. Whatever the Commission's motive, however, the point I wish to make here is that quality-of-life considerations are an essential ingredient of its best-interest standard.

Judicial Decisions: Quality of Life by Any Other Name

Of all the participants in the national debate over the ethics of terminating treatment, the courts have understandably been perhaps the most conservative, the least willing explicitly to endorse quality-of-life reasoning. In spite of the courts' evident antipathy to quality-of-life judgments, I shall argue that the landmark legal cases in this area rely, implicitly or explicitly, on qualitative criteria.

Admittedly, this thesis does not gain much support from the round of Baby Doe litigation stretching from 1981 to 1985. These cases have been dominated by an almost exclusive concern for procedure and the allocation of decision-making authority (2). Instead of reaching the substantive issues bearing on standards for nontreatment, where the quality-of-life judgments will be found, the major neonatal cases have asked: Do parents have the right to withhold life-sustaining treatments from their children (25)? Do nonrelated "pro-life" attorneys have the right to sue in defense of children (26)? And, does section 504 of the Rehabilitation Act of 1973 apply to neonatal treatment decisions (27)?

In view of the paucity of evidence in the neonatal cases themselves, which never reach the substantive issues, we might more profitably look to those landmark cases in bioethics that do confront, albeit sometimes obliquely, the problem of setting standards for life and death. We shall discover that, appearances to the contrary notwithstanding, they are firmly committed to quality-of-life reasoning.

Three well-known cases ought to provide us with a sufficiently representative sample: *In re Quinlan* (28), *Superintendent of Belchertown State School v. Saikewicz* (29), and *In re Claire C. Conroy* (30). Although quality-of-life considerations abound in these cases (or at least so I shall argue), they are partially obscured by two features common to these and other legal decisions in this area.

First, with the exception of *Conroy*, even these cases appear more concerned with determining how the incompetent person would have decided than with the problem of setting substantive standards. The operative constitutional question in both *Quinlan* and *Saikewicz* revolves around the nature and scope of a right to privacy, a right to make choices regarding intimate matters of control over one's body and sexual capacities. Thus, in *Quinlan* the explicit issue was whether Karen "could

[have] effectively decide[d] upon discontinuance of the life-support apparatus, even if it meant the prospect of natural death," were she suddenly and miraculously to become "lucid for an interval . . . and perceptive of her irreversible condition" (28: p. 663). Likewise, Judge Liacos in *Saikewicz* confirms (in even more convoluted language) that the proper constitutional test in such cases is provided by the doctrine of "substituted judgment"; that is, "the decision . . . should be that which would be made by the incompetent person, if that person were competent, but taking into account the present and future incompetency of the individual as one of the factors which would necessarily enter into the decision-making process of the competent person" (29: p. 431). Thus, the decisive issues in both cases seem to be: who should decide and what would the patient have chosen if he or she were capable of deciding?

On closer inspection, however, both *Quinlan* and *Saikewicz*, and more recently *Conroy*, exhibit unmistakable reliance on quality-of-life reasoning. In *Quinlan* the Court employs quality-of-life criteria in determining the medical conditions that permissibly trigger the invocation of privacy rights. Judge Hughes writes, "We think that the State's interest *contra* weakens and the individual's right to privacy grows as the degree of bodily invasion increases and the prognosis dims" (28: p. 664). In other words, if the treatment is painful or otherwise "invasive," and if the patient's future is grim, the right to privacy may be invoked on the patient's behalf. How grim must the prognosis be? Judge Hughes was less than perfectly clear on this point, but his conclusion seems to have been that "the focal point of decision should be the prognosis as to the reasonable possibility of return to cognitive and sapient life, as distinguished from the forced continuance of that biological vegetative existence to which Karen seems to be doomed" (28: p. 669). Thus, notwithstanding the Court's foreground fixation on the hypothetical wishes of the patient, a careful reading of *Quinlan* reveals an intriguing "subtext" devoted to determining the qualitative threshold beyond which human life need not be valiantly preserved.

In *Saikewicz* the Massachusetts Court undertook the task of discerning whether a 67-year-old man, with an IQ of 10 and a mental age of two years and eight months, would choose chemotherapy to treat his terminal leukemic condition. (The patient was terminally ill, but, since he still had possibly a year or more to live, he probably could not be placed in the category of "dying patient" required by the medical indications policy.) This attempt to discover the hypothetical wishes of a profoundly retarded individual on the meaning of life and the limits of treatment— the bioethical equivalent of squaring the circle—led Judge Liacos to an even more narrowly circumscribed inquiry into the patient's mind than we found in *Quinlan*. Still, the Saikewicz court adopted wholesale the privacy standard elaborated in *Quinlan* and went on to speculate about the conditions of Saikewicz's life and medical condition that might have prompted him to decline the chemotherapy. It noted that the patient would be subjected to suffering, the reasons for which he would never understand (29: p. 430). And in a novel gloss on the legal meaning of "best interests," which had hitherto always implied an interest in continued existence, the Court stated, "If a competent person faced with death may choose to decline treatment which not only will not cure the person but which substantially may increase suffering in exchange for a possible yet brief prolongation of life, then it cannot be said that it is always in the 'best interests' of the ward to require submission to such treatment" (29: p. 428).

Importantly, this passage reveals that the doctrine of "substituted judgment" found in *Quinlan* and *Saikewicz*, far from rising above the quality-of-life issue, merely displaces or postpones it. Even if we make the incompetent patient's hypothetical wishes the overriding question, *someone* will still have to ask *what* the patient would have wanted. Whether this someone is a court-appointed guardian (as in *Quinlan*) or a judge (as in *Saikewicz*), he will have to ask, "Given the patient's condition (her diagnosis; the benefits, if any, that she derives from living; her experience of pain and suffering; her expected longevity with and without treatment; her attitudes toward dependency, and so forth), would she want life-sustaining treatments? Once we begin to ask about the *content* of the substitute decision maker's judgment, we see that it will be grounded in quality-of-life considerations. What else is there?

Coming finally to the recently decided *Conroy* case, we find a more straightforward acknowledgment of the role of quality-of-life reasoning. Rightly abandoning the legal fiction that cases involving incompetent patients can all be resolved by means of a hypothetical and counterfactual inquiry into the patient's "true needs and wishes," the Conroy court elaborated two "best-interests" tests—a "limited-objective" and a "pure-objective" test—as necessary supplements to the already existing "subjective" test elaborated in earlier cases. The common thread uniting these two tests is an inquiry into whether "the net burdens of the patient's life with the treatment should clearly and markedly outweigh the benefits that the patient derives from life" (30: p. 1232). Here we find the clearest possible affirmation of the key tenet uniting all quality-of-life positions: that in some cases, continued life can be a greater evil than an earlier death.

A second feature of these cases (at least of *Saikewicz* and *Conroy*) that tends to obscure their commitment to a substantive quality-of-life ethic is their explicit disavowal of one particular quality-of-life standard. Whereas the trial judge in the *Saikewicz* case had considered "the quality of life possible for him even if the treatment does bring about remission," Judge Liacos of the Supreme Judicial Court countered, "[T]o the extent that this formulation equates the value of life with any measure of the quality of life, we firmly reject it" (29: p. 432). Likewise, Judge Schreiber of the New Jersey Supreme Court declined in *Conroy* "to designate a person with the authority to determine that someone else's life is not worth living simply because, to that person, the patient's 'quality of life' or value to society seems negligible" (30: p. 1233). How is it possible to reconcile these explicit refusals to indulge in quality-of-life reasoning with our earlier findings of a distinct subtext in *Saikewicz* and *Quinlan*, and with an explicit endorsement of a best-interests standard in *Conroy*?

In order to bring about this reconciliation, we will have to make a crucial distinction between two different kinds of quality-of-life judgments, which I shall refer to as "comparative" and "noncomparative" judgments. *Comparative* quality-of-life judgments state that a particular life, because of its failure to measure up to a comparative standard or norm of human well-being, is of less value than normal human lives. For example, it is sometimes said that it would be morally acceptable for a Down syndrome child with esophageal atresia to be allowed to die, on account of his mental retardation, whereas it would be unacceptable to allow an otherwise normal child to die of the same condition (31). Comparative quality-of-life judgments also allow for certain trade-offs between the welfare of so-called defective newborns and other persons. Thus, it is sometimes said that parents may decide to forego treatment if their anomalous child could reasonably be expected to place great emotional or financial burdens on the family unit or on the society that bears (part of) the cost (32).

By contrast, *noncomparative* quality-of-life judgments focus exclusively on the condition of the patient. They are based on assessments of the patient's physical and psychological condition (Is the child in pain? Is she suffering?), as well as on the likely effects of proposed medical interventions (Will prolonged treatment be ineffective in the long run? Will it be inhumane?).

With this crucial distinction in mind, we can now return to our cases. Immediately following his apparent rejection of quality-of-life reasoning, Judge Liacos tempers his criticism of the trial court judge: "Rather than reading the judge's formulation in a manner that demeans the value of the life of one who is mentally retarded, the vague, and perhaps ill-chosen, term 'quality of life' should be understood as a reference to the continuing state of pain and disorientation precipitated by the chemotherapy treatment. . . . Viewing the term in this manner, . . . we are satisfied" (29: p. 432). For his part, Judge Schreiber in *Conroy* qualifies his rejection of a quality-of-life ethic by directing his opposition to "assessments of the personal worth or social utility of another's life, or the value of that life to others" (30: pp. 1232–33). He further qualifies his position by explicitly condoning "a restricted evaluation of the nature of a patient's life in terms of pain, suffering, and possible enjoyment" (30: p. 1232) while refusing to countenance broader definitions of quality of life that would go beyond a narrow focus on pain and suffering to encompass other kinds of qualitative concerns. (This further step was endorsed in Judge Handler's partially dissenting opinion in *Conroy* [30: pp. 1244–1250].)

The way out of our apparent textual embarrassment is thus clearly marked by the distinction between comparative and noncomparative quality-of-life judgments. These qualifications by Judges Liacos and Schreiber make clear that they stand opposed, not to quality-of-life judgments as such, but rather to *comparative* judgments that would either demean the dignity and worth of impaired persons or allow their deaths for the greater good of others. Were these judges to reject all noncomparative assessments as well, they would have rejected the very basis of their own decisions, which obviously rest on quality-of-life judgments.

The relevance of these landmark termination-of-treatment cases for the issue at hand should be apparent. If judges are to advance beyond their present procedural concerns and set public standards of legally permissible nontreatment, a likely but debatable development (3), then the same principles developed in cases from *Quinlan* to *Conroy* should apply to cases involving imperiled newborns. True, the incompetence of newborns will preclude a "right to privacy" analysis focusing on the subjective wishes of the patient; but *Quinlan*'s concern for a possible return to cognitive life, *Saikewicz*'s concern for suffering that the patient will not be able to comprehend, and *Conroy*'s concern for the net burdens of continued life would all rightly apply to the imperiled newborn. If, for purposes of this argument, there were no relevant moral differences between severely impaired newborns and the gravely ill adults depicted in these cases, then it would be discriminatory to allow the latter a merciful death while insisting that all newborns receive maximally aggressive care to the very end. It is thus no small irony that the Reagan administration's various Baby Doe rules, which were supposed to implement a policy of "nondiscrimination" toward handicapped newborns, actually turn out to discriminate unfairly against them. If like cases should be treated alike, and if our society allows gravely ill and suffering adults release from the thrall of high-technology medicine, then it should do the same for its suffering children.

Current Legislation: Quality of Life in the Child Abuse Amendments of 1984

Perhaps the most telling example of the inevitability of quality-of-life judgments is provided by the Baby Doe amendments to the Child Abuse Prevention and Treatment Act of 1984 (33). This Act defined a new category of medical neglect: the withholding of "medically indicated treatment" from "disabled infants with life-threatening conditions." Although the Act requires treatment of almost all anomalous or impaired newborns, it does specify three exceptions, which provide that treatment shall *not* be required when the infant is dying, when treatment would be virtually futile and inhumane, and when the child is "chronically and irreversibly comatose."

Interestingly, the drafters of the Department of Health and Human Services' proposed regulations for this Act stated that physicians' discretion in these cases should be limited to their "reasonable medical judgment," which, they insisted, "is not to be based on subjective 'quality of life' or other abstract concepts" (34). It doesn't take a master "deconstructer" (35) to notice the glaring self-contradiction in the DHHS's stance. The exception for chronically and irreversibly comatose children obviously refers to children who cannot be categorized as "dying patients." If nontreatment is justifiable in such cases, it must be on the ground that the *quality of a permanently comatose life* does not sustain a moral obligation to treat. How then can DHHS steadfastly reject all appeals to "subjective quality of life" concepts while allowing nontreatment of manifestly nondying patients? In contrast to my analysis of the landmark court decisions, in which we successfully reconciled resort to quality-of-life reasoning with an *apparent* wholesale rejection of the concept, the contradiction within the DHHS regulations remains intractable. DHHS rejects and affirms, simultaneously and in the same respects, the acceptability of quality-of-life judgments. In order to achieve consistency, DHHS would either have to affirm the necessity of *some* quality-of-life judgments or mandate treatment of the irreversibly comatose.

Subjectivity Revisited

The scriveners at DHHS could *possibly* respond, "Oh, well, we're not really against *all* quality-of-life judgments, only *subjective* ones. The exception for the permanently comatose can thus be justified on the ground that it concerns an objectively verifiable medical condition on the lowest end of the quality of life spectrum." In spite of its initial plausibility, this sympathetic reconstruction of DHHS's position will not successfully extricate the Department from its quandary. Although permanent coma is perhaps an objectively verifiable medical condition (but, I would add, one yielding a fairly high percentage of false positive judgments), the decision to classify it as an exception to the general rule mandating treatment is anything but "medically objective." On the contrary, in deciding that the lives of permanently comatose (but nondying) infants need not be sustained, the drafters of this legislation were indisputably making a subjective judgment to the effect that life in a permanent coma is not worth living or sustaining. Thus, if anyone is "guilty" of projecting his own "subjective preferences" of the meaning of life onto the lives of severely impaired newborns, the drafters of this law in Congress and the DHHS stand justly accused. As a vitalist hardliner might put it, "How do we know that all these children would prefer death to a permanent coma?"

The final refuge for the drafters at DHHS is to maintain that, while the permanent coma exception might be subjective in the above sense, it is still objective in the sense that persuasive rational arguments can be mounted in favor of such an exception, or in the sense that the vast majority of people would not want to continue to "live" in a permanent comatose state. Staving off the charge of inconsistency on these grounds would, however, clearly amount to a Pyrrhic victory. If ethically acceptable objectivity encompasses conclusions arrived at by means of persuasive rational argument—or by means of asking what the overwhelming majority of persons would want for themselves, were they to enter a particular condition—then there would be no good reason to stop at chronic and irreversible coma. As we shall see, equally compelling arguments of both sorts can be made for nontreatment of other catastrophic impairments besides permanent coma. A fundamental problem with the Child Abuse Amendments of 1984, then, is that they clearly allow quality-of-life judgments for one condition without giving us any good reason why such reasoning may not be extended to any number of devastating conditions beyond permanent coma.

Short of espousing a rigid and untenable vitalism, quality-of-life judgments are thus possible, appropriate, and inevitable. The real question, then, asks not whether quality of life should count, but what *kind* of quality-of-life judgments should count (36).

Varieties and Levels of Quality

Rather than work out a complete taxonomy of quality-of-life judgments
here, I will close with an inquiry into three crucial questions, whose
answers point the way toward a satisfactory theory of the kinds of
qualitative judgments that ought to guide decision making in the neonatal nursery.

Quality of *Whose* Life?

The first question asks, "Whose life, whose well-being, ought to be
considered in decisions whether or not to terminate treatment on impaired newborns?" Some theorists, such as philosopher Jonathan
Glover (37) and pediatrician Raymond Duff (38), answer that in addition
to the well-being of the child in question, the happiness or well-being of
others, such as parents and siblings, ought to weigh heavily in our
deliberations. If a severely afflicted child would place great burdens on a
family, perhaps even to the point of dissolving the family unit through
divorce, such theorists contend that the parents should be allowed to
opt in favor of their own interests (or the interests of their other children) at the expense of the impaired child's life. Thus, Duff writes,
"[R]esponsible decision makers cannot avoid some 'tragic choices'—that
is, at times knowingly sacrificing, perhaps unfairly, one person's good
or life in order to protect another's" (38: p. 316). Glover makes the same
point in declaring that while infanticide must often be extremely unpleasant, "[w]here the handicap is sufficiently serious, the killing of a
baby may benefit the family to an extent that is sufficient to outweigh
the unpleasantness of the killing (or the slower process of 'not striving to
keep alive')" (37: p. 164). Thus, both Glover and Duff are prepared to
allow the second kind of comparative quality-of-life judgment described
in an earlier section: interpersonal comparisons of happiness and un-
happiness leading to trade-offs between the welfare of one person and
the welfare of others.

Several objections can be lodged against resort to this clearly utilitarian ethical principle in the neonatal context. First, even arguing within a
purely utilitarian or consequentialist framework, we would still have to
insist on a comprehensive and balanced accounting of all the relevant
consequences entailed by the child's continued life. We would have to
count, not merely the burdens that the child will impose on a family, but
also whatever benefits might accrue to a family from caring for and
living with a seriously impaired child. Advocates for nontreatment
rarely mention the actual experiences of real parents or the pleasures
that they often derive from raising an anomalous or impaired child.

A second and related problem concerns the reliability of predictions. Given the difficulty in most instances of foreseeing just how mentally or physically handicapped an infant will turn out to be, and given the equally problematic task of predicting how a family will respond to adversity, predictions to the effect that a particular child will "destroy a family" or "place undue hardship on the other children" should be received with a good measure of skepticism. While it is undoubtedly true that some severely impaired children end up placing unbearable demands and strains on parents and other siblings, it is very difficult to predict in advance which children will have this effect.

Finally, and perhaps most seriously, a utilitarian principle that allowed trade-offs between the welfare of the child and welfare of his family would most likely violate another important ethical canon, the principle of equal concern and respect (39). This principle says that all human beings (or persons) ought to be accorded, if not equal outcomes, at least equal concern and respect in the allocation of benefits and burdens. Applied to the case of impaired newborns, this principle would have us extend reasons for terminating treatment on infants to all other similarly situated persons—for example, to severely debilitated elderly patients in hospitals and nursing homes. If we are not willing to terminate life-sustaining treatment in similar circumstances for this latter group—for example, when an elderly patient suffers from serious physical and mental disabilities, thereby placing great financial and emotional demands on the family—our unwillingness would show that we are not according equal concern and respect to the interests of newborns. It would amount to applying two different moral standards to groups that do not differ in any morally relevant respects and would, in short, yield an unfair and discriminatory moral practice.

Because of these concerns for fairness and equal concern and respect for all human beings, other quality-of-life theorists have explicitly rejected all comparative trade-offs between newborns and other affected parties. Thus Richard McCormick (8), Robert Weir (20), and the President's Commission (5) allow (implicitly or explicitly) for quality-of-life reasoning, but insist that it be focused on the newborn, not on the welfare of those who might be adversely affected by the child.

Whose Definition of Quality?

Theorists who agree that quality should count can, and do, disagree on determining the point of view from which the quality of a child's life ought to be assessed. For some, the vantage point of reasonable, competent, nonhandicapped adults ought to be accorded priority in determining the boundaries of an "acceptable" quality of life. Thus, philosopher

Joseph Margolis claims that "the decision to bring to an end the lives of selected fetuses and infants . . . is *conceptually parasitic* on the decision of the competent to end their own lives" (40). That is, since newborns are incompetent and cannot judge these weighty matters for themselves, we are thrown back on the sensibilities of normal adults as the proper standard for judging the infant's quality of life. For Margolis, then, the question is, "What would most reasonable, normal adults want? Would they agree to live out this kind of life?"

This question involves the other variety of comparative quality-of-life judgment, a judgment requiring a comparison of the child's life with some normative standard of "acceptable" or "meaningful" human life. The major problem with this sort of comparison is that it seems particularly susceptible to distortion and bias. If the hypothetical question was put to them, many, if not most, normal, healthy adults might well prefer death to a life of serious mental or physical disability. But what of the child who has never known the pleasures of normalcy? From his or her perspective, such a life might well be worth living and certainly preferable to an early death (41). Once we have rejected all comparative trade-offs as violative of the principle of equal concern and respect, it would appear that the proper focus of concern is a *noncomparative* judgment bearing on the quality of the infant's life, not from the vantage point of intellectuals and athletes, but rather from the infant's own point of view. As the President's Commission concluded, "As in all surrogate decision-making, the surrogate is obligated to try to evaluate benefits and burdens from the infant's own perspective" (5: p. 219).

Even if it turns out that this perspective is extremely difficult, if not impossible, for decision makers to maintain in certain cases, the President's Commission's recommendation is valuable for two reasons. First, it can *at least* serve us well as a general rule: in most cases, we can and should ask what would be best from the infant's perspective. This will help us rule out nontreatment as an option in cases such as uncomplicated Down syndrome, where continued life is clearly a good for the child. Second, if we at least attempt to raise this question in every case, we will do much to avoid tainting our difficult moral judgments with the bias for normalcy that competent adults naturally bring to such situations.

What Quality of Life Justifies Nontreatment?

How low does a child's quality of life have to be before nontreatment becomes a morally permissible option? This is a crucial question and a great deal of ink has been spilled in trying to answer it. Rather than attempt a detailed review of this vast literature, I shall instead focus sharply (risking oversimplification) on three different kinds of answers.

Permissive Standards

Although the so-called pro-life faction couches its opposition in terms of a wholesale rejection of all forms of quality-of-life reasoning, it would be more accurate (and less inflammatory) to say that it primarily opposes a *permissive* threshold for nontreatment. According to such a standard, children born with mild to fairly serious mental or physical impairments should be allowed to die, if that is what the parents wish. Usually, the advocates of this position rely on comparative judgments of the first sort: those based on some normative standard of human existence. They say that children who will never engage in certain normal human behaviors—walking without artificial supports, enjoying normal mental activity, working for a living, or marrying—should be allowed to die (42). Thus, the principal agents in the original Bloomington (Indiana) Baby Doe case, a case involving a Down syndrome child with an esophageal defect, appeared to have concluded that the life of this retarded child would be worse than death (43).

The main problem with this standard, as the pro-life critics rightly point out, is that mere deviations from normalcy, even fairly serious ones, are not sufficient of themselves to warrant death. It is not enough to note that a child will never marry or work for a living. (Indeed, on the positive side, it might be replied that such a child will be forever spared the agony of divorce and of obnoxious bosses.) In addition, it should usually have to be shown that such a child would be better off dead. If, in spite of their defects and disabilities, children can live lives that are on the whole sufficiently satisfying from their own point of view, they should be provided with the care and treatment that they need. On this point, both the pro-life forces and the more moderate quality-of-life advocates can agree upon a common struggle against the "tyranny of the normal" (44).

Chronic, Unmitigated Pain and Suffering*

In marked contrast to nontreatment criteria based on comparative norms, the so-called "best interests of the child" standard attempts to be

---

* The following two sections (pp. 175–180) are based in part on a previously published essay, "Withholding Treatment from Baby Doe," *Milbank Memorial Fund Quarterly*, 1985;63(1):18–51. A number of paragraphs have been taken verbatim from this article, and I thank my coauthor, Professor Nancy K. Rhoden of Ohio State University, for permission to include them here.

scrupulously noncomparative. This standard, as advocated by the President's Commission and several commentators, would have us ask whether continued life is more of a burden than a benefit to any particular child. As the Commission put it, "[S]uch permanent handicaps justify a decision not to provide life-sustaining treatment only when they are so severe that continued existence would not be a net benefit to the infant" (5: p. 218). Although the Commission's wording is perhaps unfortunate (a child might cherish his life even if it doesn't yield a "net benefit"), the basic idea is sound. In spite of the fact that incompetent children's ideas of "acceptable life" are bound to vary as much as adults', we can conclude that this standard has been met in at least one type of situation. This is when the infant will suffer chronic, severe, and intractable pain. Although we usually believe that life is good or desirable, the prospect of a lifetime of unmanageable pain and suffering shatters this everyday confidence. Indeed, pain of this scope and magnitude can eclipse the child's capacity for enjoying those normal human pleasures that ordinarily predispose us to believe that life is good. Although it might be somewhat paradoxical to say that death would be a "benefit" for such a child, we *can* say that, matched against a life of unmitigated suffering, death could be viewed as the lesser of two evils. Needless to say, this is a very strict quality-of-life standard.

This approach has two distinct advantages over competing principles. In contrast to permissive quality-of-life standards, it cannot be accused of subjecting newborns either to the "tyranny of the normal" or to unfair and discriminatory trade-offs that secure the welfare of others at the expense of the child. Contrary to the position taken by the Reagan administration, nontreatment under a best-interests standard does *not* amount to "discrimination against the handicapped."

And in contrast to the pro-life medical indications principle, which merely asks if a diseased or defective *organ* can be medically improved by a corrective procedure, the best-interests principle would appropriately have us focus on the whole patient. While it may be true that doctors have no business *as doctors* in making cavalier, unfounded, and irresponsible quality-of-life judgments, it is equally true that doctors have a professional and moral responsibility to advance the good of the patient as a whole person, and that they shrink from this responsibility when they narrow their field of vision down to the functioning of discrete body parts and systems. What good does it do for a tragically impaired infant—one whose future is limited to months or a few years and whose days are marked by isolation on the respirator, by frequent seizures due to severe brain malformations and bleeding, and by one painful medical procedure after another—what good does it do for such a child to approach the impending end with surgically corrected parts and normal kidney scores? Quality-of-life judgments are thus "inevitable" in another sense: in addition to surfacing in just about every serious proposal for the care of impaired newborns, quality-of-life judgments are *ethically* inevitable if doctors are to practice fully responsible medicine (45).

Notwithstanding its initial plausibility and moral attractiveness, the best-interests standard suffers from one serious drawback: it does not apply to an entire range of situations in which nontreatment seems morally justified. What, for example, does the best-interests standard tell us in regard to the infant whose life will be very short and extremely limited but not filled with excruciating pain and suffering? If we steadfastly cleave to the child's point of view, and if the child, though catastrophically impaired, is not experiencing pain, what are we to think the child would want? An infant given the choice between an early death and five months of a blind, deaf, immobile, and profoundly retarded life—but one without severe pain—might, were he competent to decide, judge his best interests to be five months of life. Or he could believe that such a life is not worth it. We simply cannot know. Thus, the injunction to view the situation from the infant's perspective has the unfortunate effect, in the absence of unrelievable pain, of 1) giving us an impossible task (How are we to find out what the child would want?), and 2) seeming to require treatment even when it appears inappropriate or virtually futile.

Since chronic, intractable pain is not present in very many neonatal dilemmas, the best-interests standard turns out to be a morally correct, well-founded criterion that does not apply to very many cases of otherwise justifiable nontreatment. Perhaps the most telling example of this would be the application of the best-interests standard to the category of infants in permanent coma, a category already excluded from the DHHS's very strict guidelines on mandatory treatment. If we cannot say with confidence that death would clearly be in the best interest of such children—and I do not think that we can—then this standard cannot justify nontreatment even though the vast majority of reasonable, responsible adults would no doubt conclude, with the Reagan administration, that treatment is surely not mandatory in such cases. Clearly, if we wish to deal forthrightly with such cases, rather than using the child's "best interests" as a vacuous omnibus phrase connoting the permissibility of nontreatment for *whatever* reasons, then we will have to repair to a final quality-of-life threshold.

Lack of Basic Human Capacities

How, then, do we go beyond the widely endorsed best-interests principle to provide a justification for nontreatment in cases where the infant
is not in severe pain but in which decision makers simply feel that
treatment is not an act of kindness, or even of good sense, but is rather a
mindless and futile flexing of medical hardware?

The first step is to accept forthrightly that decision makers in these
cases are inevitably unable to act as agents who ascertain and implement
the patient's desires. The injunction to take the infant's perspective is
misleading, because it focuses on the unknowable and suggests that
infants in similar circumstances would have similar preferences, could
they somehow be ascertained. Moreover, it diminishes the import of
the crucial fact that the most devastatingly affected infants either will
lack the conceptual apparatus to develop preferences or will not live
long enough to develop them. Thus, this focus diverts us from the truly
important issue, which is not the infant's hypothetical desires, but
rather the sorts of lives that society wishes to labor to preserve.

Second, we can make explicit those features of the "easy" cases that
make them relatively straightforward. For example, most people would
agree that if an infant's life span is inevitably limited to days or weeks,
physicians are not obliged to extend this ill-fated life to its outer limits.
But *why* is this relatively uncontroversial? The reason, it seems, is that in
such a brief time the infant has no opportunity to develop or to do any of
the things that humans characteristically do and value. If a person cannot sufficiently partake of the human experience, as in the case of the
anencephalic infant, these days or weeks simply do not justify our medical efforts. At this fundamental level, with the dying or anencephalic
infant, we are making a quality-of-life judgment—that a brief, biological
existence bereft of human responses and joys does not, by our lights,
merit preservation. Surely, the length of time is relevant; but far more
crucial is that the infant can do and feel little during this time. Moreover,
even a lengthy life, if lived in a wholly unconscious state, is one that few
would feel must be sustained. Again, this judgment can only be based
on the belief that the quality of life without consciousness is morally
distinct from that of conscious human life. As philosopher James
Rachels puts it, "living" involves more than merely "being alive" (46).

John Paris and Richard McCormick have expressed this standard as
follows: "If [the infant's] potential [for human relationships] was simply
nonexistent or would be utterly submerged and undeveloped in the
mere struggle to survive, that young life had achieved its potential and
no longer made life-sustaining claims on our care" (47). This is especially

clear when we recognize that life-sustaining procedures are not neutral, but involve at least some degree of bodily pain and invasion. When they yield no benefit, not in the narrow sense of medically benefiting an organ, but in the broader sense of providing at least some level of experience or activity, the game is simply not worth the candle.

This harm/benefit calculus provides, I believe, ethical justification for withholding life-sustaining treatments from infants with disorders such as trisomy 13 or 18, where the life span is brief and, more important, where the ability to participate in the human experience during this short life is so radically limited. I contend that these lives, with these handicaps, are neither long enough nor full enough to require preservation by means of burdensome medical procedures. This means neither that the infants and their lives lack all value nor that we cannot love these babies and cherish them while they live. It merely means that we believe it appropriate to decide, from our own perspective (which realistically we cannot escape), that these infants' lives are so radically affected by their multiple malformations that they do not partake sufficiently of human experience to render treatment morally required.

If the standard is whether the infant has sufficient potential to live at least a minimally human life for a reasonable time span, a major problem is where to draw the line. We have made a little progress: almost all writers in this area, whatever their theory, conclude that anencephalic infants need not (and should not) be treated, while Down syndrome children should. Between these polar extremes, there is massive confusion and conflict. We have managed to give good reasons for placing infants with disorders such as trisomy 13 or 18 in a category similar to anencephalic infants. This conclusion conforms with the actual practice of neonatologists (48). (Such conformity is, of course, not a convincing moral argument, but it is a good sign.)

Other disorders that result in a radically shortened life span, or little or no ability to develop cognitively, should likewise justify withholding aggressive treatment, though infants with such disorders should be given warmth, comfort, and ordinary care. When the life would be very short (say one year or less), or, despite its length, virtually nonsentient, or, perhaps, respirator-dependent with no potential for detachment, these meager benefits are not worth it. On the other side, infants with handicaps such as Down syndrome, most cases of spina bifida, and a host of other quite serious disorders can clearly partake of enough of life's experiences to make medical treatment for them morally required.

This standard, like any that seeks a middle ground, has distressingly fuzzy edges. One can accept the principle, yet disagree violently as to whether doctors must aggressively treat the 650 or 700 gram infant with major intraventricular hemorrhages who may well die anyway, who will probably be severely or profoundly retarded if she does live, but who could possibly survive intact. Similarly, one can accept this standard yet feel hopeless confusion if a newborn with Tay-Sachs for some reason requires major medical care soon after birth. How aggressive should doctors be in treating this infant? Harder still is the case of the infant who may live for many years, but with such massive brain damage that retardation will almost surely be profound. There can be genuine disagreement as to where we draw the line and say that this life is not one that we feel should be aggressively preserved. In such instances, exclusive attention to a quality-of-life standard is not likely to yield an unambiguous, definitive resolution. When this happens, the best that conscientious, moral decision makers can do, perhaps, is to grope in the fog of uncertainty and anxiety. Nonetheless, a quality-of-life principle focused on lack of basic human capacities at least allows the debate to be centered on grounds that are intellectually honest and realistic: What do *we* think of this sort of life?

Although any adequate and honest ethic of newborn care must acknowledge the inevitability of this question, we must at the same time acknowledge the dangers involved in asking it. In marked contrast to the best-interests standard, which would allow us to make these same choices with an illusory good conscience ("We're just doing this for the sake of the child"), this full-blown quality-of-life principle requires us to make profoundly troubling choices. I suggest that intellectual honesty breeds moral unease here because this particular quality-of-life standard sanctions precisely those kinds of comparative judgment on the life of the newborn that the best-interests standard refused to allow. What the best-interests standard loses in intellectual integrity for failing to address the reality of the hardest cases, it gains in moral attractiveness. What the "lack of human capacities" standard gains in theoretical adequacy by confronting these cases, it loses in public acceptability.

The first danger is that this standard obviously involves a comparative judgment of the first sort. It openly and explicitly acknowledges that certain lives, because of their failure to measure up to a comparative standard or norm of human well-being, have less of a claim on us than other (more normal, or less blighted) lives. Although the standard of lack of human capacities presumably applies only to the most catastrophically anomalous or impaired children (those for whom the notion of "best interests" seems to have lost all or most of its meaning; those who appear to lack the basic capacities to have distinctly *human* interests), it would still have us measure these children against some sort of human norm, rather than focus exclusively on their own well-being. For any number of good reasons, we are extremely loath to admit to ourselves that some lives are "less valuable" than others on account of their lack of certain capacities. Whether we wish to put the matter this starkly or search for phrases more expressive of our abiding love and concern for such children ("Although still of inestimable value, they place less of a moral claim, or different moral claims, on society"), it remains true that this standard commits us to making momentous distinctions among members of the human community. The fact that such comparative judgments might well be practically inevitable and morally permissible does not make them any the less troubling or tragic.

Although this standard's commitment to the second variety of comparative judgment—interpersonal trade-offs of benefits and burdens—is not immediately apparent, it comes into view as soon as we raise the question of the *motivation* for withholding treatment from these "worst case" children. Supposing it is morally *permissible* to withhold life-sustaining treatment from a severely microcephalic trisomy 18 child with renal problems, why should we actually *do* so? Apart from those many instances where a proper noncomparative, patient-centered reason can be found (for example, if the proposed treatment, say dialysis, is too burdensome to the child, given her abysmal prognosis), we are left with the naked comparative judgment that continued treatment is "just not worth it." In the absence of pain and suffering for the child, we cannot meaningfully or honestly say that an early death is in the child's best interest. In such cases, then, the only possible motivation to stop treatment is based on an assessment that continued treatment would exact too great a cost in terms of parental suffering, monetary expense, or the availability of scarce health care resources. We are saying, in short, that the (very meager) benefits to the child of continued treatment are not worth the (often enormous) burdens to parents, caregivers, or society.

Notwithstanding the propriety of such comparative judgments, we do not like to think of ourselves as the sort of people who make them (49). But instead of allowing our scruples to get the upper hand, instead of simply refusing to make such interpersonal comparisons and trade-offs, we slip easily and gratefully into the false consciousness of euphemism: "extraordinary treatment," "not medically indicated," "not in the child's best interest." But if we look unflinchingly at our actual practice, we find (not surprisingly) that we *are* the kind of people who make these comparative judgments, whether or not we like to think of ourselves this way. This tension between our traditional moral ideals and the moral realities of medicine in a technological age is certainly a cause for concern. What, one wonders, will be the long-term effects of this kind of moral schizophrenia on our own self-image, both as individuals and as a society?

A "Lexical" Approach to Decision Making

We have thus discovered two distinct quality-of-life rationales for non-treatment: the standard of the child's "best interests" and the standard of a "lack of basic human capacities." The former would have us focus exclusively on the condition of the child, whereas the latter allows both comparisons of the child's level of existence with some norm of "minimally acceptable" human life and trade-offs between the child's good and that of other affected parties. Since the best-interests test sanctions nontreatment *for the sake of the child,* it poses less of a threat to our moral ideals than the other test, which requires us to make disturbing comparative judgments.

Before closing, I want to say a word about how decision makers ought to deploy these different tests. I propose that they be implemented in what economists and philosophers have called a "lexicographical" (or, more manageably, a "lexical") ordering, whereby the first principle or test must be entirely satisfied before moving on to the second (50). Applied to neonatal dilemmas, this ordering would require decision makers first to inquire about the child's best interests. They should ask, "Is this child likely to benefit from further treatment and further life?" If the answer is "Yes," then the child should be treated in spite of her physical or mental deficiencies, although we should expect strenuous debates about exactly what will count as a "benefit." If, on the other hand, we conclude that continued life would not constitute a genuine benefit to the child, if we reason that she would be "better off dead," then we should allow the child a merciful early death.

In a limited number of cases, however, this inquiry into the child's best interests will lead nowhere. We find on these occasions that the child is so lacking in basic human capacities, or perhaps her predicted longevity is so short, that it becomes problematical to describe her as having distinctly human "interests" (beyond the avoidance of pain and suffering). When, and only when, the best-interests test fails to yield any meaningful result, decision makers should then repair to the second test, based on lack of basic human capacities. This lexical ordering of principles is thus designed to avoid the *premature* and *unethical* invocation of comparative judgments upon children who can, with our help, live meaningful and happy lives.

Once the best-interests test runs out, and only then, we must apply comparative judgments in order to determine what kind of lives *we* think are worth preserving with the aid of invasive and expensive high-technology medical care. These are profoundly disturbing judgments to make and, as we have seen, members of our society go to great lengths to mask the true nature of such judgments or to deny their existence outright. Although we cannot and should not evade the anxiety that comes with making these comparative judgments, it should be some small consolation to realize that the only alternatives are an unacceptable vitalism or a strict "medical indications" policy that ignores the good of the whole patient in favor of an overweening concern for isolated lesions and malfunctioning body parts.

Concluding Remarks

Should the quality of a child's life matter to decision makers in the neonatal nursery? In this chapter, I have argued that it does, in fact, matter; and that it ought to matter. Virtually all of the proposed policy solutions to the Baby Doe dilemma incorporate a concern for the kind of life that a child will live, beyond the brute fact of physical existence, and I have tried to show that this concern is ethically justified. In some cases, it is justified by the presence of pain and suffering that eclipse the child's capacity to enjoy ordinary human goods; in other cases, it is justified by the absence of certain basic human capacities, such as the ability to relate to other people.

Beyond these specific theoretical results, I hope that this chapter will contribute to a more rational debate over quality of life. Once we get beyond simplistic condemnations of, and simplistic appeals to, an *unqualified* quality-of-life principle, we are finally in a position to see the great diversity of quality-of-life standards. Again, the proper question is not, Should quality of life count? (of course it should, because it is inescapable) but rather, Which quality of life position should we adopt?

Failing to specify *which* quality-of-life position we mean to embrace or attack can only lead to oversimplification on both sides. Thus, bald pro-life assaults on "subjective quality-of-life judgments" lump together a wide variety of quality-of-life considerations that ought to be carefully distinguished in our public debates. In doing so, they also exaggerate both the similarities between quite divergent quality-of-life positions, and the differences between some very likeminded pro-life and quality-of-life theorists. I would surmise, for example, that an avowed advocate of quality of life, such as Richard McCormick (8), has much more in common with "pro-lifer" Everett Koop (10) than with those quality-of-life theorists who deny the "personhood" of all infants (not to mention "defective" ones) and would allow the sacrifice of Down syndrome children for the happiness of their families (51). Such blanket condemnations of quality of life only serve to shore up the ideological rigidity of their proponents, while eroding the prospects for mutual understanding and reasonable compromise.

On the other hand, abstract, vague, and unqualified proposals for quality-of-life decision making lead to a different kind of oversimplification. By thoughtlessly lumping compelling ethical factors, such as unremitting pain and suffering, together with borderline retardation or mild physical disability, some advocates of quality of life would recommend a moral principle so vague in its meaning that it could easily and predictably lend itself to highly subjective and dangerous judgments for newborns. This kind of careless advocacy of quality of life tends to evoke equally careless denunciations from the other side, and wholesale advocacy is thus matched by wholesale condemnation. What we need, instead, is an honest, open, and carefully nuanced debate about the *limits* of quality-of-life reasoning.

References

1. Horan D, Delahoyte M, eds. Infanticide and the handicapped newborn. 1982.
2. Rhoden NK. Treatment dilemmas for imperiled newborns: why quality of life counts. So Cal Law Rev 1985;58(6):1283–1347.
3. Burt RA. Authorizing death for anomalous newborns. In: Milunsky A, Annas G, eds. Genetics and the law. New York: Plenum, 1976, pp 435–50.
4. Starr P. The social transformation of American medicine. New York: Basic Books, 1982.
5. President's Commission for the Study of Ethical Problems in Medicine and Biomedical and Behavioral Research. Deciding to forego life-sustaining treatment. Washington DC: U.S. Government Printing Office, 1983, chs. 1, 7.
6. Annas G. Prisoner of the ICU: the tragedy of William Bartling. Hastings Cent Rep 1984;14:28–29.
7. Fletcher J. Morals and medicine. Princeton NJ: Princeton Un Press, 1954.
8. McCormick R. To save or let die: the dilemma of modern medicine. JAMA 1974;229(2):172–76.
9. Ramsey P. Ethics at the edges of life. New Haven CT: Yale U Press, 1978.
10. Koop CE. Ethical and surgical considerations in the care of the newborn with congenital abnormalities. In: Levine C, ed, Taking sides: clashing views on controversial bio-ethical issues. Guilford CT: Dushkin, 1984.
11. Arras JD. Ethical principles for the care of imperiled newborns: toward an ethic of ambiguity. In: Murray TH, Caplan AL, eds, Which babies shall live? Humanistic dimensions of the care of imperiled newborns. Clifton NJ: Humana Press, 1985, pp 106–108.
12. Fost N. How decisions are made: a physician's view. In: Swinyard, CA, ed, Decision making and the defective newborn. Springfield IL: Charles C Thomas, 1978, pp 220–30.

13. Avery ME, Taeusch HW, eds. Schaffer's diseases of the newborn, 5th ed. Philadelphia: WB Saunders, 1984, pp 850–52.
14. Ramsey P. The Saikewicz precedent: what's good for an incompetent patient? Hastings Cent Rep 1978;8:36–42.
15. Federal Register Jan 12, 1984;49(8):1629.
16. Toulmin S. The tyranny of principles. Hastings Cent Rep 1981;11(6):31–39.
17. Fleischman A, Murray TH. Ethics committees for Infants Doe?—an alternative that deserves a chance. Hastings Cent Rep 1983;13(5).
18. Weber LJ. Who shall live? New York: Paulist Press, 1976.
19. McCormick RA. The quality of life, the sanctity of life. Hastings Cent Rep 1978;8(1):30–36.
20. Weir RF. Selective nontreatment of handicapped newborns: moral dilemmas in neonatal medicine. New York: Oxford U Press, 1984.
21. Murray TH. The final, anticlimactic rule on Baby Doe. Hastings Cent Rep 1985;15:5–9.
22. Robertson J. Legal aspects of withholding medical treatment from handicapped children. In: Doudera AE, Peters JD, eds, Legal and ethical aspects of treating critically and terminally ill patients. Ann Arbor MI: AUPHA Press, 1982, pp 213–27.
23. President's Commission for the Study of Ethical Problems in Medicine and Biomedical and Behavioral Research. Deciding to forego life-sustaining treatment. Washington DC: U.S. Government Printing Office, 1983, pp 197–229.
24. Abram M, Wolf S. Public involvement in medical ethics: a model for government action. N Engl J Med 1984;310:627.
25. In re Infant Doe, No GU8204-004A Ind Ct App Apr 12, 1982.
26. Weber v. Stony Brook Hospital, 467 NYS 2d 685.
27. United States v. University Hospital, 729 F.2d 144 (2d Cir 1984).
28. In the matter of Karen Quinlan, 355 A.2d 647, 70 NJ 10 (1976).
29. Superintendent of Belchertown State School v. Saikewicz, Mass., 370 N.E.2d 417 (1977).
30. In the matter of Claire Conroy, 486 A.2d 1209 (NJ 1985).
31. Shaw A. Dilemmas of 'informed consent' in children. N Engl J Med 1973;289:885–90.
32. Strong C. Defective infants and their impact on families: ethical and legal considerations. Law Med Health Care, Sept 1983:168–81.
33. U.S. House of Representatives. Amendments to child abuse prevention and treatment act. Congressional Record—House. (Sept 9, 1984):9805–18.
34. Child abuse and neglect prevention and treatment program, proposed rule. Federal Register Dec 10, 1984;49(238):48160.
35. Campbell C. The tyranny of the Yale critics. New York Times Mag Feb 9, 1986:20 ff.
36. Reich WT. Quality of life and defective newborn children: an ethical analysis. In: Swinyard CA, ed, Decision making and the defective newborn. Springfield IL: Charles C Thomas, 1978, pp 489–511.
37. Glover J. Causing death and saving lives. Harmondsworth, England: Penguin, 1977, ch. 12.
38. Duff RS. Counseling families and deciding care of severely defective children. Pediatrics 1981;67(3):316.
39. Dworkin R. Justice and rights. In: Taking rights seriously. Cambridge MA: Harvard U Press, 1977, p. 180.

40. Margolis J. Human life: its worth and bringing it to an end. In: Kohl M, ed, Infanticide and the value of life. Buffalo: Prometheus, 1978, pp 180–91.

41. Robertson J. Involuntary euthanasia of defective newborns. Stanford Law Rev 1975;27:254.

42. Lorber J. Ethical concepts in the treatment of myelomeningocele. In: Swinyard C, ed, Decision making and the defective newborn. Springfield IL: Charles C Thomas, 1978.

43. Rebone H. "Minimal quality of life": why parents, courts chose Infant Doe's death. Hosp Prog, June 1982;63:10.

44. Fiedler LA. The tyranny of the normal. In: Murray TH, Caplan AL, eds, Which babies shall live? Clifton NJ: Humana Press, 1985, pp 151–59.

45. Angell M. Handicapped children: Baby Doe and Uncle Sam. N Engl J Med 1983;309(11):659–61.

46. Rachels J. Euthanasia. Oxford: Oxford U Press, 1985.

47. Paris J, McCormick RA. Saving defective infants: options for life and death. America Mag 1983;148(16):313–17.

48. Levin BW. Consensus and controversy in the treatment of catastrophically ill newborns: report of a survey. In: Murray TH, Caplan AL, eds, Which babies shall live? Clifton NJ: Humana Press, 1985, pp 169–207.

49. Calabresi G, Bobbitt P. Tragic choices. New York: Norton, 1978.

50. Rawls J. A theory of justice. Cambridge MA: Harvard U Press, 1971, p 43.

51. Singer P. Euthanasia for defective infants. In: Practical ethics. Cambridge, England: Cambridge U Press, 1979, pp 131–38.

7

The Principle 'Patients Come First' and Its Implications for Parent Participation in Decisions

CARSON STRONG

Decisions concerning selective nontreatment of impaired newborns are among the most controversial in medical ethics. The focus of this chapter will be the question of who should make these decisions. This is usually referred to as the *procedural* issue. Since the procedural issue is closely related to the *substantive* question of what ethical principles should be followed in making these choices—and in my view cannot be discussed apart from it—the substantive issue will also be addressed. Traditionally, selective nontreatment decisions have been made by the parents, with the advice and counsel of the infant's physician. In the wake of controversy over the 1982 "Baby Doe" case in Bloomington, Indiana, the federal government challenged this traditional approach by assuming a regulatory role in these decisions (1). This challenge appears to rest on two beliefs. First, it is held that nontreatment decisions should be based solely on the interests of the infant. Second, since there is often a conflict of interest between infant and family, parents are not considered the best decision makers for the purpose of securing the infant's well-being. The latest federal regulations, implementing the Child Abuse and Neglect Amendments of 1984, are the product of a hard-fought political struggle involving organized medicine, the right-to-life lobby, and advocacy groups for the disabled, among others (2). Thus, the question of who should make these decisions is no longer academic, but has entered the public arena.

Given the growing concern over the procedural issue, we might ask what the alternatives are. What are the policy options from which we might choose in deciding who is to make these decisions? While there is a variety of forms the alternatives can take, I believe the ones being seriously considered can be divided into three broad categories. First, there is the traditional approach, in which the decisions are made by the parents and physician. For purposes of this discussion, this approach can be understood as encompassing forms of interaction between physician and parents involving varying degrees of influence by the physician. Second, the decisions could be made by ethics committees at the institution caring for the patient. Committees could formulate rules to be followed, and selected cases could be brought before committees prospectively for resolution. Third, the decisions could be stipulated by regulatory agencies through the enforcement of rules. Presumably, such decision making could originate at local or state agencies, as well as federal. Combined forms are possible, of course, in which some decisions are made by one of these parties and some by another.

Other decision makers have been suggested, including physicians acting alone and the courts. However, these approaches do not appear feasible at present. To eliminate parental consent entirely, in lieu of the physician's decision, would be considered unacceptable by most because of its infringement of parental responsibility. Oversight of all decisions by courts would be unduly cumbersome. In general, courts lack sufficient familiarity with the clinical setting to unilaterally formulate comprehensive and helpful policies. Court involvement is more workable when it is limited to the occasional case involving needed clarifications of law or disagreements between parents, physicians, and hospitals.

It will facilitate discussion if we consider the three basic options mentioned above: parents and physicians, ethics committees, and regulatory agencies. A major way in which these basic options differ is in the degree to which the decision maker is removed from the situation being resolved. Parents and physicians are closest to the clinical situations in which the need for decision-making arises. Ethics committees, on the other hand, are somewhat removed from those situations, and regulatory agencies are even more remote from them.

At present, decision making by regulatory agency has largely supplanted the traditional approach. U.S. Department of Health and Human Services (DHHS) regulations require that life-sustaining procedures be provided unless one of the following conditions is met: the infant is irreversibly comatose; the treatment would merely prolong dying, not be effective in correcting all of the infant's life-threatening conditions, or otherwise be futile in terms of the survival of the infant; or the treatment would be virtually futile and would be inhumane. Furthermore, medical hydration and nutrition must always be provided, even when one or more of these conditions is present (2). Thus, the discretion of parents and physicians is limited to judgments concerning whether any of the three conditions is met. This discretion includes, with regard to the second condition, judgments that there are uncorrectable conditions that will cause death in the near future. The third condition involves judgments that treatment would be highly unlikely to prevent death in the near future and that the treatment itself either has significant medical contraindications or involves pain and suffering that outweigh its very slight potential benefits. Needless to say, this is a very narrowly defined area of discretion.

I want to explore the question of which of these three types of policy options ought to be used. Thus, I want to examine this challenge to the traditional approach. For this purpose, I shall accept the assumption that the interests of the infant should take priority in these treatment decisions.* I shall argue that even if we grant this assumption to challengers to the traditional approach, parents and physicians are nevertheless the best decision makers. Then I want to explore the meaning of the principle that the health professional's primary obligation is to the patient, with particular attention to conflicts between the interests of infant and family. Finally, I shall discuss what I think are the *real* problems with the traditional approach, and areas of needed improvement.

The Traditional Approach

In our culture parents have a moral responsibility to provide for the care and nurture of their children. At a basic level this involves making sure that one's children receive needed food, clothing, shelter, and medical care. However, this parental responsibility also includes seeing to it that one's children are properly educated, that moral guidance is provided, and in general that their well-being is promoted. Within this realm of responsibility parents are permitted a certain amount of discretion concerning how these needs are to be met. Thus, parents have considerable latitude in the choice of schools, the assignment of chores, and the inculcation of religious beliefs, to mention just a few examples. This area of discretion is perhaps not well-defined, but nevertheless it is real and important. Several reasons can be given in support of there being such an area of discretion. First, there is great diversity of opinion concerning proper ways of providing for the well-being of children. There is no way of doing it that is self-evidently the best approach. Second, the autonomy of individuals is a value of great importance. Respect for autonomy requires that we respect the decisions of parents concerning family life. Third, the well-being of families should be promoted. This suggests that interferences with parental decision making that are likely to cause harm to families should be avoided. Moreover, since families are usually in

---

* The question of whether family interests *should* sometimes be permitted to override important interests of the infant is a separate issue, and has been discussed elsewhere (3).

the best position to decide what will promote the interests of their members, such decisions should generally be left to the families themselves.

Not only are parents responsible for decisions within this area of discretion, but they have a right to make these decisions. If parents did not have a right to be the decision maker and others could legitimately make these choices without consulting the parents, then the claim that parents are responsible for these decisions would be meaningless. This right to decision making has limits, of course. When parental decisions are likely to result in harm to a child, the state may intervene, as in cases of treatment refusal on religious grounds. While the law recognizes limits to parental rights, it embodies a strong presumption in favor of family autonomy against state intervention. Reasons supporting this presumption were well-expressed by the President's Commission for the Study of Ethical Problems in Medicine and Biomedical and Behavioral Research:

Families are very important units in society. Not only do they provide the setting in which children are raised, but the interdependence of family members is an important support and means of expression for adults as well. Americans have traditionally been reluctant to intrude upon the functioning of families, both because doing so would be difficult and because it would destroy some of the value of the family, which seems to need privacy and discretion to maintain its significance (4: p. 215).

Several landmark cases illustrate this strong presumption. The seminal case was *Meyer v. Nebraska*, in which the Supreme Court held that the "liberty" guarantee of the Fourteenth Amendment "without doubt . . . denotes . . . the right of the individual . . . to marry, establish a home and bring up children" (5: p. 399). Applying this principle, the court upheld the right of the parents to have their children taught the German language. In *Wisconsin v. Yoder* the court held that compulsory education laws were not applicable to the parents of Amish children who had completed eight years of public school education. Because secondary education in public schools influences children in ways that would undermine the integration of Amish children into their religious community, the court decided that compulsory education beyond eighth grade would violate the traditional interest of parents with regard to the religious upbringing of children. The alternative education offered within the Amish community would satisfy the state's interest in protecting children from ignorance, according to the court (6). Similarly, in cases involving parental decisions concerning medical treatment, courts interfere with parental autonomy only when it is outweighed by considerations of large magnitude, such as death or other serious harm to the child (7).

The traditional approach in which parents were permitted to make the decisions concerning impaired newborns appeared reasonable, since all the reasons supporting an area of discretion supported the inclusion of these decisions in that area. First, there is great controversy concerning what is in the best interests of the infants in these cases, and often there are no clear answers. Second, because these decisions have great potential to affect the course of family members' lives, to remove them from parental hands would significantly undermine family autonomy. Third, it was not unusual for families to suffer significant harms in the process of caring for impaired infants, due to inadequate financial, professional, and institutional support services. This suggested that the state should not intervene in these decisions—in the absence of adequate governmental and community support—in order to avoid harming families.

Traditionally, parents have not made all the decisions for congenitally impaired infants. Physicians have played a large role and have usually had the power to make certain decisions themselves and to bring parents into the decision-making process when appropriate. Good arguments can be given for the view that certain decisions should be left to the physician. Specifically, there are many situations in which it is reasonably clear that treatment is the best course for the purpose of promoting the infant's interests. Even when there is evidence that the infant might be impaired, as in cases of perinatal asphyxia, there is often considerable uncertainty about whether the infant will in fact be handicapped and no evidence that continued life will cause suffering. In such circumstances the best interests of the infant require aggressive treatment, at least until evidence accumulates that the prognosis is poor. In such cases the physician has a clear professional obligation to treat and need not know the parents' wishes in order to decide what should be done. We might say, therefore, that an acceptable way for physicians and parents to share decision making within the framework of the traditional approach would be as follows: The physician ought to allow parents to participate *unless* professional duties or other moral considerations dictate, independently of parental wishes, what the decision ought to be. Of course, even when physicians are justified in making unilateral decisions, parents should be kept informed.

The Patient's Best Interests

Before weighing the pros and cons of the policy options, it will be helpful to discuss one of the important substantive issues: What principles should be followed in order to promote the best interests of the infant? The answer to this question has implications for the issue of who should make the decisions, as we shall see. Two main views can be identified concerning this substantive question. According to the first view, actual or potential cognitive impairments of infants should not be regarded as a morally relevant consideration in deciding what is best for them. To consider such factors morally pertinent is to fail to respect the patient's full status of personhood, according to this view. Decisions are to be made by considering what would be an appropriate choice for any person, regardless of handicap. This view is illustrated in an early version of DHHS regulations, which stated that withholding life-preserving treatment from infants with congenital anomalies constituted discrimination against the handicapped. DHHS claimed that "It is only when non-medical considerations, such as subjective judgments that an unrelated handicap makes a person's life not worth living, are interjected in the decision-making process" that discrimination occurs (8). Others have advocated this viewpoint, including Paul Ramsey, who states, "[T]he standard for letting die must be the same for the normal child as for the defective child. If an operation to remove a bowel obstruction is indicated to save the life of a normal infant, it is also the indicated treatment of a mongoloid infant" (9: p. 192). Similarly, Edwin Healy makes the following comment in discussing the use of artificial respiration for an infant with hydrocephalus: "Every infant, no matter how grossly deformed he may be, is a human being and as such has the same right to life as that which is enjoyed by a perfectly normal child. Whatever a physician would be obliged to do for a normal child, he must do for this hydrocephalic" (10: p. 89).

According to the second view, on the other hand, a substantially diminished potential for cognitive development can sometimes be morally pertinent to judgments about the infant's welfare. On this view life has value insofar as it enables one to have experiences that are valuable to oneself. Decisions are to be made by considering whether infants will have such experiences to sufficient degree to make continued life in their interests.

A similar conflict of views arises concerning withholding medical nutrition and hydration. According to the first view, the prognosis for survival and cognitive functioning is not relevant to the question of whether nutrition and water should be provided. Since their provision is not only life-preserving but a symbolic expression of care and concern, to withhold them might be interpreted as showing a lack of concern for patients and a failure to respect their status as persons. Thus, food and water should always be provided. This view, too, was asserted in earlier DHHS regulations forbidding the withholding of medical nutrition and hydration: "[T]he basic provision of nourishment, fluids, and routine nursing care is a fundamental matter of human dignity, not an option for medical judgment. Even if a handicapped infant faces imminent and unavoidable death, no health care provider should take it upon itself to cause death by starvation or dehydration" (8: p. 30852). According to the second view, the prognosis for survival and cognitive development can be relevant to decisions concerning fluids and nutrition in some cases. If the prognosis is sufficiently poor, it might be concluded that all life-prolonging medical procedures, including provision of hydration and nutrition, should be discontinued. Although such a decision would depend on a judgment that withholding fluids and nutrition would not cause discomfort to the patient in question, the second view leaves open the possibility that such judgments are sometimes reasonable.

In contrasting these two views, we can see that they emphasize different ethical considerations. The first view focuses on the objective of respecting the patient's status as a person. It seeks to promote the equality of rights and interests of all persons, regardless of degree of handicap. It advocates, as a method of promoting such equality, the following of certain rules that aim to protect the personhood of patients. Examples are

The lives of persons should be preserved.

Food and water should not be withheld from persons.

The second view emphasizes that decisions should take account of the well-being of patients in addition to their rights and status as persons. It asserts that decisions should be individualized, based on the facts of the particular situation, rather than based on fixed rules. I shall refer to the first view as the *inviolateness-of-persons* approach, with the understanding that the rules in question are designed to protect the inviolateness of persons. I shall call the second approach a *beneficence-based* view, to reflect its emphasis on protecting the well-being of persons.

Both of these views have strengths and weaknesses. A major advantage of the inviolateness-of-persons approach is its relative ease of application in clinical practice. Given a set of definite rules, the application of them is often straightforward, avoiding the task of weighing conflicting ethical considerations in the context of each unique case. For example, such an approach can eliminate agonizing decisions over provision of fluids and nutrition. It can also reduce the number of difficult decisions about provision of other life-support measures. Another strength is that it helps ensure that patients are not treated as though they lack the full status of personhood. Such protection seems important, given the various incidents that have been reported in which the moral status of patients has been given questionable or inadequate attention (11–13). A major weakness of this rule-based approach, however, is the difficulty in devising a set of rules that will yield plausible conclusions in all cases. This approach underestimates the great variety and complexity of clinical situations. It is likely that any set of rules would, in some cases, produce conclusions that are wrong. The current regulations, for example, sometimes yield conclusions that are at odds with our intuitions. An illustration involves care of anencephalic infants. Since the regulations require that fluids and nutrition always be provided (2), this requirement extends to anencephalics. Since these infants are often unable to suck or swallow, artificial nutrition and hydration must be provided in order to follow the rule. However, artificial feeding would not benefit such infants. Lacking a cortical brain, they do not experience pain, thirst, or hunger. Moreover, providing food would only prolong an inevitable dying process.

A second main weakness is that the rule-oriented approach fails to acknowledge the gray areas in which there is controversy about what would promote the patient's interests. The examples include infants with fatal genetic diseases, such as trisomy 18 syndrome. Approximately 30 percent of infants with this condition die by age one month, and 50 percent by two months. The 10 percent who survive one year are invariably severely mentally handicapped (14). Sometimes these infants have additional life-threatening conditions at birth, and the question of whether the infant's interests would be promoted in providing treatment for immediately threatening conditions is a difficult one. The issue becomes even more controversial when we consider specific treatments. One case I encountered involved a trisomy 18 infant who had an esophageal atresia. Also, the level of bilirubin in the blood was rising due to immature liver function. Excessive levels of bilirubin can cause death or brain damage. Several life-prolonging procedures were being provided or considered, including surgical correction of the esophageal atresia, parenteral fluids and nutrition, and exchange transfusions to lower the bilirubin level. There was considerable controversy and doubt concerning which of these procedures should be provided in order to promote the child's well-being.

Another type of case that falls in the gray area involves infants with severe brain injury due to perinatal hypoxia. An example is an infant who was delivered by emergency cesarean birth for fetal distress at 28 weeks' gestational age. His distress was believed to be due to an infection *in utero* caused by rupture of the amniotic membranes. The infant had severe bradycardia and Apgar scores of 0, 1, and 1 at one, five, and 10 minutes after birth. Resuscitative efforts produced little response initially, but after an intracardiac injection of epinephrine the infant was resuscitated, taken to the intensive care nursery, and given respirator therapy. A diagnosis of pneumonia and septicemia was made. These infections were treated, but seizures soon began and the infant exhibited no spontaneous movement. A computerized tomography scan revealed areas of hemorrhage in the brain. Several weeks later there was no improvement in the infant's neurological condition. The prolonged absence of physical movement indicated severe brain damage. This might be a child who would always be bedridden. In this case, too, there was doubt about whether continued respirator therapy would be in the patient's interests.

The difficulty in deciding gray-area cases is often compounded by certain typical features of clinical situations involving impaired newborns. One of these is uncertainty concerning the infant's subjective states of experience. For example, in the case involving the infant with trisomy 18, one of the issues concerned what procedures would provide comfort or prevent suffering. Would excessive bilirubin levels cause pain or suffering? Would withholding fluids and nutrition cause the infant discomfort? The answers were unknown, since it is frequently difficult to ascertain what the neonatal patient is experiencing. Another factor is uncertainty about the infant's prognosis. In the case of the infant who suffered perinatal hypoxia, for example, there was uncertainty concerning the degree to which the infant would be handicapped in the long run. The possibility that the child would not be severely impaired suggested that treatment might be in his best interests. On the other hand, it was highly probable that he would be seriously handicapped, suggesting that treatment might provide little benefit. The rule-based approach does not take adequate account of these uncertainties.

In some gray-area cases, treatment as well as nontreatment might be permissible. If either is permissible, a rule requiring treatment might be objectionable. Since there are values in addition to the interests of the infant that are worth promoting in these gray-area cases, such as the right of parents to participate in decisions, the inviolateness-of-persons approach can be criticized insofar as it thwarts those values. Both the diversity of clinical situations and the frequent occurrence of gray-area cases suggest that it is important to be able to individualize decisions. Moreover, since the factors creating diversity and uncertainty are clinical ones, it is important that the decisions be made by someone close to the clinical situation, so that these factors can be taken into account.

The main strength of the beneficence-based approach is that it avoids those conclusions of the inviolateness-of-persons view that are at odds with our intuitions. By taking into consideration the unique features of each case, the beneficence-based approach can better serve the needs of

particular patients. A main weakness is that this approach is often relatively difficult to apply in clinical practice. Deciding when the quality of
patient's lives is so poor that continued treatment would not be in their
interests involves difficult judgments, complicated by several factors.
These factors include the clinical uncertainties mentioned above concerning prognosis and the patient's subjective states. In addition, there
is a disagreement over the criteria that should be used in assessing the
patient's well-being.

Two main questions can be raised concerning the criteria issue. First,
what are the criteria supposed to be criteria *of?* Two types of answers to
this question can be given. According to one view, life-preserving treatment should be withheld only when it is reasonable to believe that the
patient would not have a *meaningful* life if survival occurs. Various views
concerning what constitutes a meaningful life have been put forward,
including the ability to interact with others (15) and the ability to be self-
supporting and live independently (16). A second view maintains that
life-preserving treatment promotes the infant's interests only if continued life would *benefit* the infant. The main difference between these
views is that two different comparisons are involved. The first view
makes an implicit comparison between the patient's expected quality of
life and a norm of human ability. When that quality of life is sufficiently
below the norm, the patient's life is considered not to be a meaningful
one. The second view compares the infant's expected quality of life with
the absence of life. It asks whether continued life would be better for the
child than death itself. If the positive experiences are likely to outweigh
the negative ones (pain and suffering), then continued life is viewed as
benefiting the patient, on balance.

The second view appears to be the preferable one, for two reasons.
First, the meaningful-life view disregards the possibility that a life might
benefit the one who lives it even though it is below some norm of
human capacity. From the perspective of the impaired individual, even
relatively simply pleasures and activities might make continued life better than death. Second, assertions about whether a life is meaningful
appear close to, and might be indistinguishable from, judgments about
the *worth* of a life as viewed by another, as opposed to its value to the
one who lives it.

The second question concerns what criteria should be used in making quality-of-life comparisons. Given the framework of the second view
discussed above, various criteria are possible. According to one view, if
pleasurable experiences occur with sufficient frequency and duration to
outweigh the infant's painful experiences, then continued life benefits
the infant (17). Thus, pleasure and pain are the important criteria, on

this view. Other criteria, however, take into account the ways in which cognitive abilities confer benefit to a person's life. The absence of such abilities would reduce the extent to which a life benefits the one who lives it. These might include the ability to experience the affective and cognitive aspects of interpersonal relationships. Another criterion would be the capacity for self-awareness, as opposed to simple consciousness. Yet another is the ability to formulate and carry out personal plans. Some might claim that a favorable balance of pleasures and pains, in the absence of one or more of these cognitive abilities, is not sufficient to make continued life beneficial (18). The resolution of this issue concerning quality-of-life criteria is an important problem facing the beneficence-based approach.

In weighing the strengths and weaknesses of the inviolateness-of-persons and beneficence-based approaches, it seems reasonable to conclude that the beneficence-based view is better suited for application to clinical situations. Although there are difficulties in applying the beneficence-based approach, these difficulties reflect the genuine controversy and uncertainty that surrounds these decisions. In this sense, the beneficence-based view is more true to life than the inviolateness-of-persons view is. Moreover, it is preferable because it does not commit us to the implausible conclusions of the inviolateness-of-persons approach. This suggests that we should strive to find a reasonable way to apply the beneficence-based view, rather than adopt the alternative.

Who Should Make the Decisions?

Let us consider the pros and cons of each main policy option, beginning with decision making by regulatory agencies. As stated above, this approach involves the enforcement of substantive principles by governmental bodies. This raises the question concerning which of the two main views regarding substantive principles should be enforced. It is evident that the only way a regulatory agency *could* specify the decisions to be made in particular cases is by adopting a rule-based approach. The beneficence-based approach involves individualized decisions, made by weighing the factors affecting infant well-being in each case. Therefore, an adoption of it by a regulatory agency would require that decision making be relinquished to others more directly involved in the specific situations, such as committees or family and physician. Thus, it is no surprise that those instances in which regulatory decision making has been implemented—namely, the various Baby Doe regulations—the enforced principles have consisted of the inviolateness-of-persons approach. In evaluating the regulatory option, therefore, we need to keep in mind the pros and cons of the inviolateness-of-persons approach.

One advantage of the regulatory option derives from the inviolateness-of-persons approach. To the extent that its enforced rules are unambiguous, their application in the clinical setting will be relatively straightforward. Another strength is that all hospitals would be subject to the same rules, thereby promoting a principle of justice according to which similar cases should be treated similarly. In addition, this option provides a mechanism for preventing serious abuses resulting from undue influence of the interests of family, physician, or hospital. However, the weaknesses of this option include those of the inviolateness-of-persons approach. Specifically, the regulatory approach does not allow for individualized decisions based on the facts of each particular case. This can result in a failure to consider the needs of individual infants properly and yields conclusions at odds with our intuitions. Another major problem with this option is its intrusion into an area of decision making that traditionally has been a family responsibility.

There are various ways in which regulatory bodies can influence decisions, of course. Instead of dictating decisions, regulations might establish a framework of general principles to guide decision making. (For example, it might be required that decisions be made within the framework of choosing what is best for the infant.) Alternatively, regulations might simply specify procedures to be followed. These types of influence, however, do not come under the category we have discussed, in which choices are specified by the regulatory agency. They would presumably be versions of the other two options.

Decision making by committee is an option with several potential strengths. Committees, like regulatory bodies, can constitute a mechanism for preventing undue influence of the interests of family or physician. They could also resolve disputes between family and physician, in some cases at least, avoiding expensive and cumbersome legal proceedings. Depending on their composition, committees might be able to offer expertise concerning matters relevant to the decision. This might include knowledge about the law, or the availability of community resources to assist families caring for handicapped children. Decision making by committee might also promote the goal of taking into account all the relevant ethical considerations. In spite of these possible advantages, there are serious questions about whether ethics committees in the role of decision maker would work effectively in practice. To the extent that committees are removed from actual clinical situations, they would lack firsthand knowledge of the cases being decided, a fact that could diminish the quality of decisions. In addition, clinical decisions must often be made without great delay, thereby precluding prospective committee deliberation. Another practical consideration is whether the benefits provided by an institutional ethics committee would be regarded by institutional officers as worth the costs, including expenditure of time and effort by personnel. If a committee is not considered worth the effort, there might be institutional pressures to minimize its activities. Another major concern is that committee decision making, like the regulatory approach, would intrude into areas of family responsibility.

Of course, committees might function in useful ways other than making decisions. They could serve in an advisory capacity, making nonbinding recommendations to physicians and families. In this role committees would enhance the decision-making process by identifying options, addressing legal questions, clarifying alternative ethical viewpoints, and helping to ensure that all relevant information is considered. Given the difficulties in decision making discussed above, due to clinical uncertainties and differing ethical views, the process of decision making could probably be enhanced by committees acting in an advisory role. Ethics committees could also fulfill an educational function, providing information to families and health care providers. Since, in these roles, committees would not be making decisions, such involvement would presumably be part of an approach in which choices are made by parents and physicians or regulatory bodies.

The third option, in which decisions are made by families and physicians, has important advantages. First, it involves decision making by those closest to the actual clinical situation. This allows the decision makers to have a firsthand understanding of the unique features of the particular case, so that decisions can be appropriately individualized. This seems essential to the process of trying to identify what is best for each patient. Second, this approach preserves an important area of family responsibility. The argument supporting family participation in decisions is particularly strong in gray-area cases. As stated above, there are good reasons supporting the view that parents should have the opportunity to make decisions unless it is clear, independently of parental wishes, what the decision ought to be. Therefore, in the gray-areas in which it is not clear what would be best for the infant, parents should be permitted to make the decisions. It is their responsibility and they have a right to participate. A potential weakness of this option is that the interests of family and physician might have undue influence on the decisions in some cases. However, it seems to be widely conceded that abuses would occur only rarely.* As a way of preventing such abuses,

---

* In its regulatory impact analysis, the DHHS acknowledges that the number of cases of unjustifiable withholding of treatment is small (2). A similar assessment has been made by others (19, 20).

regulatory bodies could establish a framework for decision making according to which the infant's interests are to be primary, while allowing families and physicians to interpret how this is to be implemented in specific cases. This would counteract, although perhaps not eliminate, tendencies to let other interests take priority. Another weakness is that physicians and parents sometimes lack knowledge needed for well-thought-out decisions. This deficiency could perhaps be overcome to some extent by the use of ethics committees serving an advisory role.

Consideration of the strengths and weaknesses of these three options suggests that decision making by parents and physicians is the best approach. An assumption of those who have challenged the traditional approach—that the infant's interests are best served if someone other than parents and physician makes the decisions—does not withstand critical scrutiny. Decision making by regulatory bodies is unsatisfactory because it is restricted to an inviolateness-of-persons approach, which yields implausible conclusions and fails to consider the individualized needs of patients. Ethics committees are questionable decision makers because they are removed from the actual clinical situation and are too cumbersome to make those decisions of a relatively urgent nature. Furthermore, decision making by regulatory agencies and committees intrudes into areas of family responsibility, an invasion that is especially unwarranted in gray-area cases.

Duty to Infant and Family

We have assumed, for the sake of argument, that decisions for impaired newborns should be based strictly on the best interests of the child. It has been argued that, given that objective, the best policy is to permit parents and physicians to make the decisions. When they are the decision makers and the general framework is that of giving primacy to the infant's interests, another important question arises for health professionals: What does it mean to say that the health professional's primary obligation is to the patient? This is a question that needs to be explored in order to better understand the health professional's duties when the interests of infant and family conflict.

Most physicians would agree with the proposition that their primary obligations are owed to the patient. The frequent reference to this principle in the codes and writings of physicians is evidence of its wide acceptance. The World Medical Association, for example, adopted a pledge known as the Declaration of Geneva, which states: "The health of my patient will be my first consideration" (21: p. 109). The editor of the *New England Journal of Medicine* recently stated that "a physician's obligation is primarily to help his patient, and not the patient's parents or next of kin or legal guardian" (22: p. 109). Similarly, neonatologist Mildred Stahlman has written: "I believe, as the Hippocratic oath states, that the physician's first responsibility is to act in the best interests of his patient, then in the interests of the parents, and finally in the interests of society, in that order" (23: p. 519).

The question arises as to why the physician's duty to the patient should take precedence over the interests of the patient's family. Physicians have written relatively little about this question, despite the importance they give to this principle. One approach to this question is suggested by Jonsen and Jameton in a recent essay (24). In their discussion of the social responsibilities of physicians, they attempt to ground the physician's ethical obligations on a conception of the function and role of physicians. In applying this approach to the issue we are now considering, we would need to identify the main functions associated with the role of physician. Most would probably agree that the primary function of the physician has traditionally been to help the sick by applying knowledge and skill in diagnosing and treating illness. Although contemporary physicians carry out various activities, including elective abortions, cosmetic surgeries, artificial inseminations, and promotion of wellness, among others, a central feature of the physician's role continues to be treating the sick. As stated in the American College of Physicians Ethics Manual: "The primary goals of the physician are to relieve suffering, prevent untimely death, and improve the health of the patient while maintaining the dignity of the person. All the physician's acts toward these ends stem from the physician-patient relationship. Ethical behavior toward patients is to a great extent that which furthers these goals and strengthens the physician-patient relationship" (25: p. 131).

The primary duties associated with the role thus described can be conceived as those which would promote the carrying out of these functions. This suggests that the physician's primary duties include, as stated by Jonsen and Jameton, exercising due care in diagnosing and treating, and having a personal concern for the patient's interests. Other duties include respecting the rights of the patient, with particular attention to those rights the protection of which advance the objectives of the doctor-patient relationship, such as rights to informed consent and confidentiality. Such patient-centered duties, on this view, should be regarded as uppermost by physicians.

Thus, there are good reasons for the view that physicians' primary obligations are those toward their patients. However, there are at least two ways one can interpret the concept that the duties to patient are primary. On one hand, it can be held to imply that the interests of the patient should *always* take priority over the interests of the family. A number of arguments can be put forward in support of this position. As Jonsen and Jameton point out, because physicians in general are known to espouse the principle of putting patients first, patients assume that physicians will act according to that principle. Because this expectation is created, physicians have an obligation to carry through. Another argument is based on the utilitarian consideration that people will, in general, be more likely to seek health care if they trust doctors. It is claimed, furthermore, that people are more likely to trust doctors if it is perceived that doctors always put the interests of patients first. In addition, a relationship of trust has therapeutic advantages, in that it reduces anxiety and enhances compliance. Another argument, based on prudence, might go as follows: Society should require physicians to put the interests of incompetent patients first, since any of us might some day become incompetent patients. In addition, it might be argued that there is an implied agreement with the incompetent patient's family to do what is best for the patient.

According to the second view, the interests of the family are permitted to take priority over the patient's interests in some cases, provided the encroachment of the patient's interests is relatively small and the harm to the family thereby prevented is great. This view is consistent with the idea that the physician's primary obligations are to the patient, for several reasons. First, when the potential harms to patient and family are roughly equal, this view gives priority to the patient. Second, this view never permits a serious sacrifice of the patient's interests for the sake of the family, although it does permit serious harm to the family for the patient's sake. Third, this view gives priority to the patient in the great majority of cases, since conditions in which a small invasion of the patient's interests can prevent severe harm to the family occur in only a small percentage of situations.

The second view gives greater emphasis to professional obligations to family members. It seems quite clear that health professionals have obligations to families. An illustration is the obligation to respond to the needs of family members for emotional support when a patient is seriously ill or dying. The basis of this duty is the principle of beneficence, the family's need in a time of crisis, and the ability of health professionals to provide such support. There are various ways in which physicians and other health providers can give emotional support: by carefully explaining the patient's medical condition, treatment, and prognosis; by reassuring the family that everything reasonable is being done to help the patient; showing concern for the family as well as the patient; and listening to the concerns expressed by the family. Another professional obligation is to assist families who assume the task of providing special care for patients. Family needs can be especially great when the patient has handicaps. Assistance might involve informing families of available community resources, referring the family to specialists, and giving advice about problems. According to the second view, when interests are in conflict a balancing of the duties to patient and family is allowed, within limits. Minor infringements of the patient's interests are permitted to avoid serious harm to the family.

The question arises, of course, as to which of these two views is more reasonable. Certain considerations suggest that the second view is to be preferred. To begin, there is an adequate reply that can be made to each of the arguments supporting the first view. None of those arguments supports the position that an infant comes first even if great harm is thereby caused to the family. Thus, none of them do what they purport—to show that the patient's interests should *always* come first. The implicit agreement with the patient referred to by Jonsen and Jameton, as well as the therapeutic advantage, do not apply in the case of newborn patients. Neither does the prudential argument, since none of us will be neonates again. In addition, the utilitarian goal of encouraging parents to seek medical care for their children would seem to be promoted as well if not better by alternative principles, such as: Give priority to the infant's interests unless doing so would cause great harm to the family, in which case do what the parents wish. (I am not advocating this principle, but citing it in order to point out the shortcomings of the utilitarian argument.) Thus, the utilitarian argument does not establish that the interests of patients should always come first. Moreover, concerning any implied agreement with an incompetent patient's family, it is doubtful that parents generally agree, whether explicitly or implicitly, that the physician is to do what is best for the infant regardless of the degree of harm that might cause the family.

Additional support for the second view derives from the fact that it is more in line with our moral intuitions. Consider the occasional situation in which it becomes evident that continued efforts to save a premature infant will not be successful. One such case I encountered involved parents who, from the time of the birth, had difficulty accepting the possibility that their premature daughter might die. In conversations with the physician they stated firm beliefs that their daughter was going to live, and kept urging that everything possible be done for her. When it became clear to the doctors that the child was dying, a discussion occurred on rounds concerning what should be done. One approach would be to immediately discontinue the life-prolonging respirator treatment. There was no obligation to the patient to continue the respirator therapy since it would be futile. Furthermore, although it was not clear what the infant was experiencing, continued treatment might prolong any discomforts she was feeling, including any associated with tracheal intubation. However, abrupt cessation of treatment would probably be emotionally traumatic for the parents. Another approach would be to delay the withdrawal of treatment while the health care team tried to help the family be more emotionally prepared for this event. This psychological support would mainly consist of helping the parents understand and accept the reality of the situation. The poor prognosis and futility of treatment could be emphasized in a compassionate, supportive manner. After giving the family a day or two to adjust to this bad news, the treatments could be stopped. Although this approach might prolong discomfort of the infant, it would help prevent serious harm to the family associated with the shock of learning that their daughter's treatment was being terminated. In spite of this slight compromise of the patient's interests, a delay for the family's sake appeared to be the right approach. However, the principle of always doing what is best for the patient would suggest stopping treatment at once, to avoid the possibility of prolonging even minor suffering of the infant. These various considerations favor the second interpretation of the principle that the health professional's primary obligations are those toward the patient.

Improving the Process of Decision Making

In arguing that the policy best promoting the well-being of infants involves decision making by parents and physicians, I do not mean to imply that there are no problems with this approach. However, I suggest that the main shortcomings are not the ones identified by right-to-life groups who have criticized this traditional approach. While their criticism has focused on what they consider to be unethical withholding of treatment, the question of when it is ethical to withhold treatment is highly controversial, and cases of unjustifiable withholding appear rare. The real problems, rather, lie in the ways that information and decision making are shared between physicians and parents. Specifically, it seems that the areas of needed improvement include the three discussed below.

First, there is a tendency of neonatologists to pursue aggressive treatment without involving parents in the decisions, even in situations in which parents should be permitted to participate. Having observed decision making in an intensive care nursery for several years, I have found that during nursery rounds it is not unusual for medical staff to avoid the question of withholding treatment. Discussions often focus on numbers and technical data, with little explicit mention of the patient's overall well-being. Sometimes a brain-damaged infant stops breathing or develops bradycardia and is resuscitated with oxygen or a respirator with no prior attempt to have a discussion with the parents in anticipation of such events. Various types of physician behavior have the effect of minimizing parental involvement in decisions. For one thing, physicians sometimes do not tell parents what they know about the infant's possible handicap, including brain damage due to hypoxia. A reason often given for this is based on the fact that frequently there is uncertainty about whether a child will be handicapped, as well as the degree of impairment. If potential handicaps that the parents learn about do not materialize, it is claimed, then they will have been worried needlessly. I have heard a neonatologist say that the term 'brain damage' should never be used in the nursery, since there might be some parent within earshot. Presumably, terms that parents would not understand should be used, such as "neurological impairment." This doctor went on to explain that when parents hear about brain damage, they assume the worst concerning their own baby.

Another common physician behavior is being too optimistic in discussing an infant's condition with the parents. An example is given by Rottman, who conducted a study of the interaction between neonatologists and parents of low-birthweight infants. Delivery of a baby girl at 27 weeks' gestational age was precipitated by surgical treatment of her mother's ruptured appendix. During the first few months of the infant's life the problems associated with her prematurity were played down to the point of being described as normal. Afterward the mother stated, "It all sounded so easy—just leave your baby with us for X number of months while she matures and we'll deliver your finished, perfect child at the end. Little did I realize that seven months later she would still be oxygen dependent and unable to leave the hospital." The child subsequently developed bronchopulmonary dysplasia, a debilitating chronic lung disease caused by respirator therapy. As Rottman put it, "The reassurance they had initially 'that lung tissue can regenerate itself' proved to be optimistic and misleading" (26).

There are several paternalistic arguments one frequently hears in the intensive care nursery supporting the view that parents should be excluded from life-or-death decisions. These are based on the emotional turmoil parents experience when they learn their baby is seriously ill. Although the response varies from one parent to the next, some reactions are typical. The situation is usually perceived by parents as a crisis, characterized by grief over the loss of the normal baby that was expected (27). Feelings of guilt and failure often are present because parents suspect that the infant's problems are somehow their fault. The grieving process has been described in terms of stages, beginning with shock and followed by denial, sadness, and anger (28). One argument is referred to as *the guilt rationale*. It holds that parents should not be allowed to participate in life-or-death decisions because they might suffer intense guilt if they decide to let their baby die or keep alive an infant who turns out to be seriously handicapped (29). *The anxiety rationale* is based on the idea that weighing the pros and cons of withdrawing treatment is almost certain to cause great stress and anxiety for parents (30). According to *the inability to decide logically rationale,* parents in states of shock or denial have difficulty assimilating information about their child's condition. It is claimed that their emotional condition and lack of knowledge interfere with their ability to think clearly and make rational decisions (23).

However, none of these arguments withstands critical scrutiny. The guilt rationale overlooks guilt the parents might later experience when they realize they did not fulfill their responsibilities to make these important decisions. The anxiety rationale also fails to consider harms that can occur to parents when the seriousness of the child's condition is not divulged. This can include emotional shock upon later receiving news for which they were not properly prepared, such as learning about serious handicaps or the death of their child. The inability to decide logically rationale underestimates the strengths of parents. Some clinicians have confirmed that, despite initial shock and denial, most parents can be brought to have a satisfactory understanding of the situation and can make reasonable decisions (31). Counseling and support from the health professionals, through repeated meetings and repetition of the basic facts, can facilitate this process.

A second shortcoming occurs in situations in which it is reasonably clear what should be done to promote the interests of the infant, and hence there is no need for parents to make a treatment decision: even in these circumstances parents are often not adequately informed. Bogdan and colleagues studied patterns of communication between intensive care nursery physicians and parents (32). Those authors reported that although physicians believed that they told parents everything, they actually imparted information selectively, based on a classification of parents according to their level of comprehension and compliance with physicians' expectations. Parents who asked too many questions were considered troublesome and were referred to the senior physician. The "good parents" are those who are compliant and intelligent. The well-known account by the Stinsons, who describe the six months of treatment and eventual death of their premature son Andrew, explains that they were regarded as "difficult parents," in part because they disagreed with the physicians' philosophy of aggressive treatment. When they subsequently obtained the medical records of their child, they learned that there was much they had not been told:

Andrew's bronchopulmonary dysplasia had first been noted nearly two months before we were informed of it. He had had more infections than had been reported to us, had been on more drugs of a seemingly experimental nature than we knew of and had bone problems more severe and fractures more numerous than we have been told. We found out that Andrew had developed an iatrogenic cleft palate. We learned for the first time about the gangrene that had developed in his infected leg and of the tissue and muscle that had been cut away down to the bone; we had been told only that Andrew had an abscess which had been drained and which had "healed nicely" (33: p. 68).

Even when parents are not "difficult" there is often inadequate communication. Rottman describes a number of instances in which parents were surprised or angered to learn that treatments had been carried out without an attempt to inform them, and reports that parents generally are given limited access to medical information (26).

A third shortcoming is that pediatricians and obstetricians sometimes provide very inadequate counseling to parents of handicapped children (20). Sometimes this is due to not keeping up-to-date concerning the prognosis of infants with congenital handicaps. For example, there is a tendency to overestimate the percentage of Down syndrome patients who are severely or profoundly mentally retarded. To consider another example, it is sometimes not explained that almost every child with Down syndrome has some chronic medical problem, such as speech difficulties, hearing loss, recurrent upper respiratory infections, or constipation. Another problem that has been reported is that physicians are sometimes inappropriately optimistic or pessimistic in their counseling of parents (20). Also, physicians occasionally are not well-informed about the availability of community resources to assist families caring for handicapped children.

I do not mean to suggest that these various shortcomings are universal. No doubt, there is a fair number of physicians who inform, counsel, and share decisions with parents in a sensitive, nonpaternalistic manner. However, in a matter as important as treatment of impaired newborns we should keep open a critical eye and strive for improvements in the process of decision making. The main weakness of the traditional approach is not the abuse of parental discretion. Rather, the problem lies in just the opposite direction—the shortcomings in physician-parent interaction discussed above.

References

1. Fost N. Putting hospitals on notice. Hastings Cent Rep 1982;12:5–8.
2. U.S. Department of Health and Human Services. Child abuse and neglect prevention and treatment program. Federal Register 1985;50:14878–901.
3. Strong C. The neonatologist's duty to patient and parents. Hastings Cent Rep 1984;14:10–16.
4. President's Commission for the Study of Ethical Problems in Medicine and Biomedical and Behavioral Research. Deciding to forego life-sustaining treatment. Washington DC: U.S. Government Printing Office, 1983, p 215.
5. Meyer v. Nebraska, 262 U.S. 390 (1923).
6. Wisconsin v. Yoder, 406 U.S. 205 (1972).
7. Veatch RM. Death, dying and the biological revolution. New Haven CT: Yale U Press, 1976, p 131.
8. U.S. Department of Health and Human Services. Nondiscrimination on the basis of handicap relating to health care for handicapped infants. Federal Register 1983;48:30846–52.
9. Ramsey P. Ethics at the edges of life. New Haven CT: Yale U Press, 1978, p 192.
10. Healy EF. Medical ethics. Chicago: Loyola U Press, 1956, p 89.
11. Jones JH. Bad blood: the Tuskegee syphilis experiment. New York: Free Press, 1981.
12. New York University School of Medicine, Student Council. Ethical issues in human experimentation: the case of Willowbrook State Hospital research. New York: Urban Affairs Health Program, New York University Medical Center, 1973.
13. Veatch RM. Experimental pregnancy. Hastings Cent Rep 1971;1:2–3.
14. Smith W. Recognizable patterns of human malformation, 3d ed. Philadelphia: WB Saunders, 1982, p 15.
15. McCormick R. To save or let die: the dilemma of modern medicine. JAMA 1974;229:172–76.
16. Lorber J. Spina bifida cystica: results of treatment of 270 consecutive cases with criteria for selection for the future. Arch Dis Child 1972;47:854–73.
17. Brandt R. Defective newborns and the morality of termination. In: Kohl M, ed, Infanticide and the value of life. Buffalo: Prometheus Books, 1978, pp 46–57.
18. Smith HM. What makes a life worth saving? (letter) Hastings Cent Rep 1984;14:48.
19. Moskop JC, Saldanha RL. The Baby Doe rule: still a threat. Hastings Cent Rep 1986;16:8–14.
20. Elkins TE, Crutcher D, Spinnato J, Anderson GD, Dilts PV Jr. Baby Doe: is there really a problem? Obstet Gynec 1985;65:492–95.
21. World Medical Association. Declaration of Geneva. World Med J 1956;3(suppl):10–12.
22. Relman A. Treating children without parental consent. In: Basson M, ed, Troubling problems in medical ethics. New York: Alan R Liss, 1981:109.
23. Stahlman M. Ethical dilemmas in perinatal medicine. J Pediatr 1979;94:516–20.

24. Jonsen A, Jameton A. Social and political responsibilities of physicians. J Med Philos 1977;2:376–400.
25. American College of Physicians, Ad Hoc Committee on Medical Ethics. American College of Physicians Ethics Manual. Ann Intern Med 1984;101:129–37.
26. Unpublished observations.
27. Solnit AJ, Stark M. Mourning and the birth of a defective child. Psychoanal Study Child 1961;16:523–37.
28. Drotar D, Baskiewicz A, Irvin N, Kennell J, Klaus M. The adaptation of parents to the birth of an infant with a congenital malformation: a hypothetical model. Pediatrics 1975;56:710–17.
29. Avery GB. Neonatology: pathophysiology and management of the newborn. Philadelphia: Lippincott, 1975, p 12.
30. Fost N. Counseling families who have a child with a severe congenital anomaly. Pediatrics 1981;67:321–24.
31. Kelsey B. Which infants should live? Who should decide? Hastings Cent Rep 1975;5:5–8.
32. Bogdan RB, Brown MA, Foster SB. Be honest but not cruel: staff/parent communication on a neonatal intensive care unit. Human Organization 1982;41:6–16.
33. Stinson R, Stinson P. On the death of a baby. Atlantic Monthly, July 1979:64–72.

V

Perinatal Policy in a Pluralistic Society

8

Perinatal Ethics in Anthropological Perspective

ROBERT A. HAHN

The ethical principles and ethical theories that have developed in Western civilization are expressed in Western language and concepts, based on Western understandings of human nature, the environment and cosmos; they are motivated by values that are also distinctively Western. Anthropological recognition that other, non-Western societies maintain very different concepts, understandings, and values leads directly to several questions about the foundations, reference, and scope of the Western ethics with which we in the West are most familiar.

1.   Do these same ethical principles (about what it is right to do and not to do) hold within non-Western societies? Are Western theories (about the bases of ethical principles, the kinds of ethical agents, the nature of ethical concepts) also valid for non-Western societies? The very notion of "ethics" itself and the place of ethics in relation, for example, to religion and social life, may be very different in different societies. Assuming these societies have developed fields of thought roughly equivalent to our conception of ethics, are their principles and theories commensurate or compatible with ours, or do they contradict them? Can we know these other principles and theories, and, if so, how?

2.   Even within Western society, there has been great diversity of cult and culture, each version embracing radically different views of the world and the proper life. Do the ethical principles and theories that have evolved in Western society minister to, foster, or tolerate these differences? Or do they ignore or homogenize and destroy them?

3.   If these Western principles and theories are found not to be applicable to or in non-Western societies (or distinctive populations within a Western society), in what sense should they be regarded as "ethics" rather than more narrowly as "Western ethics"? If Western "ethics" is thus culture-bound and parochial, is a universal ethics possible, and if so what might it look like? (Questions such as these arise not

The author is grateful for the collaboration of Marjorie Muecke, CRN, Ph.D., on related projects, and for the comments of Brigitte Jordan, Ph.D., anthropological midwife to this vital issue.

only for ethics but for other branches of philosophy as well, for aesthetics, and perhaps also for the philosophy of mind, of language, of science, and for metaphysics—ontology and epistemology.)

This chapter addresses these ethical queries as they arise in regard to fundamental issues of birth and its surrounding events. In such an inquiry, as in anthropological inquiry more generally, it is important to define the problem as broadly as possible in order to allow for cross-cultural variation. Overreliance on our expectations may lead us to "discover" what we expect. We are not likely to find or learn from differences where we do not look.

Defining birth itself is the first issue. Is the temporal beginning of the perinatal period the "glint in someone's eye," or is the birth in question one in a long sequence of rebirths whose course is cosmically ordered and personally altered in prior lives? Does the perinatal period end when the infant has been "delivered," or when he or she becomes a "person," however personhood may be thought to be constituted and achieved? While this chapter will focus on the time between the events surrounding conception and those following birth, this restriction should be regarded as somewhat arbitrary, as the introduction to a much broader topic which may address the concerns of obstetric, primary care, midwifery, and other clinical practitioners in the settings of Western medicine.

I begin by presenting sketches of the ethical theories, principles, and practices of birth in four U.S. ethnic groups (Navaho, Chinese, black, and white) and in one profession centrally engaged in these matters (Western medicine, and especially obstetrics). My goal is to raise the issues of ethical differences and compatibilities within U.S. society, and to explore the possibility of a transcultural perinatal ethics.

It should be noted that I have not engaged in primary research on the subject. Nor are the topics I discuss always central to the research of others on which my cultural sketches are based. I am more concerned to mark the presence of an issue than to define its details. For each of the groups I portray, I synthesize the reports of diverse observers on topics that bear on the issue in question. It should also be noted that, even if valid, cultural sketches are guides—formulations of cultural rules and standards—which do not necessarily predict what any one person in the given society will do; rather they describe central expectations, rationales, and partial explanations.

Since their disciplinary origins in the nineteenth century, anthropologists have been interested in the organization of societies into groups, and in the ways in which societal segments interact, realign, and perpetuate themselves. It is thus somewhat surprising that the issue of birth has been rarely considered until the last two decades (1–4). The anthropological predominance of male observers and male informants in the field may have led to this neglect; the same interaction is likely to have led not only to neglect of the topic but to bias in what has been reported (5, 6). It is probably the recently increased consciousness of issues regarded as women's which accounts for the growth of cross-cultural concerns. Anthropologists have discussed related topics: the contributions of males, females, other agents, and virgin birth in the formation of fetus and infant (1, 7); the significance of twins (8); abortion (9); "pollution" by reproductive products—menstrual, seminal, and parturient (5); and the "couvade" (2) in which men either deliberately restrict their activity during the pregnancy of their spouses or, unwittingly, develop increased (and often pregnancy-like, pseudocyesis) symptoms during their spouse's pregnancy. Mead and Newton (2) reviewed what is reported in the ethnographic literature as well as methodological shortcomings in this research, and they proposed expansions.

There is good reason to expect great ethical variation across cultural boundaries. Let us say that a society's ethics formulates the society's notions about *who should do what to whom (or to what) under what circumstances.* The society's ethics will presumably justify these principles on the basis of some higher scheme of desirable order. Principles of ethics must themselves rest on other concepts: concepts of 1) the kinds of agents there are who can or cannot be responsible, 2) the capacities of these agents to act or forbear from acting and the achievement and the loss of these capacities, 3) the modes of causality and influence by which agents effect their certain consequences, 4) the nature of choice and fate in this causal system, 5) the values and goals which are sought in ethical action, and 6) the principles, forces, or beings which justify these values and goals. We must know, for example, if and when a conceptus is thought to attain a status which makes its control or elimination immoral. We must also know at what stage a human achieves status as, say, a person who may hence be expected to be morally responsible; and we must know under what conditions these capacities are lost, and how responsibility is then redistributed. From these premises follow reasonable assignments of credit and blame. Such metaphysical and eschatological concepts are controversial and difficult to ascertain even within Western civilization. They are perhaps more difficult yet to ascertain across cultural boundaries (10). Nevertheless, anthropological evidence suggests enormous variation on these matters from society to society.

In the cultural sketches below I cover a broad range of topics about the ethics of birth, insofar as information is available. I explore notions of causality and responsibility as they apply in the course of perinatal

events. More specifically, I attempt to document general notions of gender roles, sexuality, reproduction, and the "life cycle" in the greater
scheme of things. In more detail I examine ideas, values, and practices
regarding conception, including contraception, fertility and infertility,
sterilization, abortion, implantation, adoption, and legitimacy. Regarding pregnancy I examine values and understandings of pregnancy and
birth as pathological or healthy, natural or supernatural, of male and
female responsibility, the couvade, diagnosis, termination, and care for
mother and fetus. On the issue of birth itself, I describe desired attendants and the "division of labor," and the agent (mother or physician/
midwife) said (or thought) to "deliver" the infant. Finally, regarding the
infant, I look at ideas about personhood and identity, infanticide, notions of parental responsibility and that of others, and desired goals.
(Though I do not deal with it here, the issue of abuse touches several
facets of the perinatal subject—especially rape, spouse abuse, and child
abuse; see, for example [11].) The ideal contents of these cultural accounts could be displayed in tables such as Table 8.1. On each substantive topic, we would want to know what principles of cause and effect
obtain, what personal and other agents are involved, what ends are
desired, what is the division of labor and responsibility, and what are
the rewards and sanctions for compliance and violation.

Navaho

In the Navaho world, not only humans themselves, but a variety of
supernatural entities and forces are believed to interact to influence the
course of events, including those of humans, their health and suffering.
Indeed, the term "supernatural" misleads, since what may appear supernatural to us is felt, among the Navaho, to pervade inextricably the
natural world and the life of humans within it (12). Traditional Navaho
thought disperses the notion of causality widely in the cosmos (13).
Causality is said to be thought of in deterministic, nonteleological terms;
mistakes are regarded as inevitable (thus without blame), and stoicism is
a common stance (14). The Navaho universe is said to be full of hazardous forces and beings. Ladd (14) claims that danger and fear are the
major reasons given to justify ethical prescriptions; the prescriptions are
sanctioned by the visitations of cosmic harm in the form of sickness and
other misfortune. The central ethical concept in Navaho thought is *ba-
hadzid*, which literally means "for it there is reverence or fear" (14: p.
237).

Knowledge and power are also achieved through close engagement,
through interaction with cosmic agents and possession by cosmic forces.

Table 8.1. The Ideal Contents of an Ethnography of Childbirth and Perinatal Ethics

	Agents, Personnel, Other Forces	Causal Effects	Desired Goals	Division of Labor, Responsibility	Sanctions, Rewards
Sex					
Gender role					
Reproduction					
Sexuality					
Personhood					
Ontogeny					
Privacy					
Pollution					
Conception					
Contraception					
In-/fertility					
Eugenics					
Sterilization					
Abortion					
Legitimacy					
Implantation					
Diagnosis					
Pregnancy					
Diagnosis					
Un-/healthy					
Super-/natural					
M/F responsibility					
Couvade					
Care					
Birth					
Attendants					
Division of labor					
Care					
Infancy					
Personhood					
Parental care					
Adoption					

Healing, too, requires cosmic encounter, and is thus in itself a hazardous activity (15). (Western physicians are thought to question and examine patients excessively because they lack such sources of knowledge and power.) Ethics and morality are not clearly distinguished from cosmology and religion, politics and law, medicine, economics, and knowledge in general. The rights of persons and their ethical obligations derive from their roles in cosmic process.

Navaho society is matrilineal: one's membership in clans, which effect major social division, is defined by the membership of one's mother. Incest is thought to be a cause of insanity or infertility; one is required to marry into clans other than one's own. Male and female children thus have distinctive values in Navaho society; primacy may be placed on females for lineage continuity (16, 17). Marriage is regarded as a prerequisite for childbearing; adultery is regarded as theft (14). Postmarital residence is matrilocal, that is, in the home of the wife's mother. These principles of Navaho social organization largely define members' relationships and major responsibilities. For example, "A man must not look at his mother-in-law and she must not look at him"; the consequence of such a look is that "You will not be very strong and your body will be weak all over," and that you "will go blind" (14: p. 230).

Woman's role is traditionally the perpetuation and maintenance of her clan. Menarche is sacred and is celebrated in a special ceremony that recalls the cosmological origins and continuing role of menstruation and clan reproduction (18). Children are desired also for their help in the chores of daily life and for the assistance they give in their parents' old age. "Children should take care of their parents" (14: p. 254).

Traditional Navaho had an average of seven children. Motherhood is regarded as "the only way to be" (19). Infertility is socially devalued. (Only a quarter of traditional Navaho women were found to use any method of contraception; contraception may be regarded as ethical insofar as it does not interfere with one's responsibility to clan and cosmos.) Abortion is practiced for "illegitimate" and unwanted pregnancies, but it is frowned upon. Infanticide was traditionally known but uncommon, and also condemned (17).

Menses are regarded with great ambivalence (19). On the one hand they are recognized as the source of fertility. Menstruation is thought of as the most fertile period of the menstrual cycle (14, 19). When united with semen during menstruation, menstrual blood is thought to form the fetus; thus menses cease following conception. Continuing menses consequently indicate infertility, and are held to be highly polluting and dangerous. Menstruating women must thus avoid ceremonial involvement, and may endanger the health of the fields, livestock, sick people, children, and men (who may be crippled following intercourse with them). Menstrual products must be properly disposed of since they may contaminate others or provide vehicles for witchcraft. Failure to observe menstrual taboos thus threatens cosmic order. Violation is said to result in difficult birth. Sexuality, too, is polluting, and abstinence is required during ceremonial periods. Husbands are also expected to restrict certain activities during the pregnancies of their wives; failure to do so is thought to result in specific congenital anomalies. Modesty is a powerful behavioral principle which may be significant in medical, gynecological, and obstetric settings. Navaho say that "A man who looks upon the organs of a woman will be struck by lightning," and "if anyone sees up your legs they will go blind" (14: p. 234).

The event of birth among the Navaho is traditionally a social and public event as well as a spiritual and religious one. "Anyone who comes and lends moral support is invited to stay and partake of what food is available" (quoted in 20: p. 153). Husband and healing singers are common attendants. Many informants say the dead fetus has no ghost. At birth, the Holy People are thought to send wind into the infant, and thus to give the infant a mind (17). The attachment of the infant's soul is thought to be indicated by its first laugh (15). This attachment is crucial since the vagaries of the soul significantly affect a person's health, sickness, knowledge, and other powers. The kind of "wind" which predominates in a person determines his or her characteristics; ethical delict may be fatalistically ascribed to these winds, and personal responsibility is thus diminished. Children (and drunks) are thought to be morally incompetent and to require severe instruction (14). Parents are also thought to be responsible for the physical shaping of their infants, by pressure massage following birth. While parents, especially mothers, are held responsible for the care of infants and children, young children are also ascribed a certain autonomy in health care; they may independently refuse treatment (15).

A principle of egalitarian, nonauthoritative "talking it over" is said to pervade Navaho interaction (14). Ladd describes Navaho attitudes toward humanity as a "non-competitive individualism." He also characterizes the Navaho ethical system as "egoistic" and "prudentialist," meaning "not only that the system is rationalistic but that it is oriented to the welfare of the individual agent" (14: p. 213). Crime and other antisocial behavior are thought to result from loss of mind, or craziness (14). Interdependence rather than independence is the dominant value in social relations; in a broader sense, Navaho seek the maintenance of harmony in their cosmos and among its beings. In medical settings, Western medicine will be accepted for its benefits of symptomatic relief while traditional medicine will be maintained as well for its ministry to underlying disorder. Navaho have not sought detailed information about medical problems and procedures, but they have been offended by the failure of medical practitioners to respect their ways (21). Navaho are said to highly respect one another's opinions and practices.

Chinese

Traditional Chinese also place human life within a framework of entities and forces that pervade the cosmos; there is no categorical distinction between natural and supernatural, human and nonhuman, spirit. In such a system of beliefs and values, individual autonomy may be neither a valued objective nor even a clear notion. Fox and Swazey write that at the heart of Chinese social relationships and ethics lies a notion of "the individual as a social community" (22: p. 339).

Knowledge and power (or capacity) ensue following proper attuning with cosmic forces; they may be sought, moreover, not in order to dominate nature, but to attain greater balance. While Western medicine achieves diagnoses by elimination ("ruling out"), traditional Chinese medicine is said to proceed by elaboration (23). Epistemological foundations are quite different (24); Unschuld (25) describes Chinese epistemology as "modest." Several key elements (earth, wood, fire, and others), their qualities (for example, "hot" and "cold"), and processes (yin and yang) interact to effect harmony and disharmony at different times and places, and in different beings. Health and sickness are direct products of these confluent events. Unschuld (25) argues both that traditional Chinese thought has lost its sway in the twentieth century, and that, in contrast to the common (Western) view of Chinese medicine, ontological theories (which conceive of disease as the localized invasion by concrete things) have always been popular alongside more systemic, holistic theories.

Pregnancy and birth, as imbalances in cosmic forces, are thus regarded as pathological occurrences (26), though they are also recognized as necessary for the achievement of the essential goal of ancestral continuity. The ancestors are venerable and active agents in current life. They must be continuously propitiated; failure to do so is thought to result in sickness and other misfortune.

Traditional Chinese society was divided into large clans and patrilineages within clans; that is, the dominant social groupings were defined by descent from common male ancestors. A rule of exogamy, requiring marriage with a person from a clan or patrilineage different from one's own, was once strongly maintained (27); rules such as these defined incest, propriety, legitimacy, and responsibility. Postmarital residence was patrilocal, that is, requiring the bride to live in the household of her husband.

Traditional marriages were arranged, and bride and groom had little to say about the affair. Love is said not to be a prominent part of their relationship; indeed relationships with husband and mother-in-law are commonly harsh. The bride is regarded essentially as the means of producing male heirs who would perpetuate the patrilineage. Reproduction may thus be felt to be a cosmic and religious duty (28). Female infants have been little valued in the Chinese tradition, sometimes sold for labor and as future brides, sometimes killed at birth. A wife's status in a new and alien household is established only when she produces a male heir. If she fails in this goal, her husband might take other wives or concubines. During the course of her life, a woman is expected to show obedience to a sequence of three males: to her father before her marriage, to her husband's family after marriage, and to her son in widowhood. Marriage was assumed to be a prerequisite to sexual relations and reproduction, but the children of concubines are also regarded as legitimate heirs to the patrilineage.

Sex was traditionally regarded in cosmic terms, as a means of reproduction, but also as a source of loss of vital yang essence; sex might thus severely weaken and sicken males (29) as well as contaminate sacred processes and relations with ancestors and supernatural beings. Menstruation and the blood at birth are also regarded with great ambivalence. Menstrual blood is thought to be the substantial source of the fetus whose development is simply initiated by insemination. But at the same time, menstrual and partum blood are regarded as highly polluting, disrupting religious and ancestral communication, and threatening the health of all who are contaminated, especially infants, men, and the infirm.

Sexual abstinence is regarded as unnatural, but Chinese are said to have no moral objection to contraception, sterilization, or abortion (30); only rare informants take fatalistic attitudes toward the consequences of sexual intercourse (30). With high infant mortality and a preference for male infants, contraception and abortion may have been traditionally rare. The principal objection to abortion and contraception is their hazard to the woman's health.

The fetal soul, *Thai Sin*, is thought to be loosely attached to the infant at conception, and to stay only until about four months following birth. Until its attachment, the soul wanders and is subject to harm affecting the fetus and infant as well (31). The child is thought to develop to moral competence only if it has "heavenly instinct"; otherwise, cosmological imbalance may lead to sickness and disharmony requiring some form of redress (32).

The mother is held responsible for premature birth and for various birth defects (27). A pregnant woman may be said to be a "four-eyed person." The month following birth, however, is thought to be more dangerous, and to require more precaution and care than the prenatal period of pregnancy. The health of both mother and infant are delicate, so that activity, diet, and other exposures must be appropriately restricted. Birth products, placenta and fluid, are thought to bear spiritual connection to the infant; they must be delicately handled and properly disposed of. Moreover, the mother and her bodily effluents are a threat to others as well, and must be isolated and avoided. Female obstetricians and other attendants are greatly preferred not only for reasons of modesty but also to avoid the contamination of males by the birth process (26).

The 'proper attitudes and behavior of infants and children are regarded as the direct responsibility of both parents; parents feel responsible when children behave improperly. Social manners are carefully inculcated—cooperation, patience, and self-control (27). Independence is not a great virtue; will is socially subjugated; emotional and self-expression are greatly constrained. Respect for education and professional achievement may lead Chinese to accept (or to appear to accept) medical prescriptions without good understanding or questioning (27). While Chinese Americans and non-American Chinese also (29) are reported to readily accept Western medicine, they also maintain traditional medical beliefs and practices (33). Western medicine may be thought of as a one-shot operation, traditional medicine as a means of restoring underlying disorder (26, 34).

White Middle-Class Americans

Reproduction and birth are perhaps the most sensitive and volatile social issues in contemporary popular politics in the United States. It is thus unfortunate, and perhaps surprising, that we know very little about the world views—the basic understandings and values—which inform and motivate debate and action in the perinatal arena. With rare exception (i.e., 35), literature on this confrontation takes the form of polemic or superficial survey rather than more objective, in-depth analysis. It is far easier to learn about the world view of perinatology among the Navaho than among middle-class U.S. whites.

Diversity of views on medical ethics has a long history in the Western world. Carrick (36) has elegantly formulated the range and sources of attitudes, values, and practices found in Greek and Roman times. It should be noted that the Greeks and Romans believed most births did not require trained medical attendants, and that at most attended births, midwives rather than physicians were present. Nevertheless, Greek and

Roman ethics are commonly inferred from the doctrines of physicians of the time. It is commonly assumed that the Hippocratic Oath, which bound physicians to secrecy among themselves and forbade them from administering euthanasia, abortions, and perhaps contraception, was the prevalent ethic. Carrick shows that the body of "Hippocratic" writings (only loosely ascribed to Hippocrates) was only partly of Pythagorean origin (prescribing the sanctity of human life, including the fetus). The Hippocratic writings were not consistent, however; some texts, for example, prescribed contraceptive formulas. Carrick suggests that many Greek and Roman physicians did not take the Hippocratic Oath, and may not even have been aware of its existence. Moreover, contraception, abortion, and infanticide were common in Greek and Roman society. Abortion and contraception were often aided by physicians, who were not regulated by the state or otherwise forbidden in these practices. These practices were strongly opposed by the Pythagoreans, but were otherwise justified by several philosophers, including Plato and Aristotle. Plato, in fact, enjoined infanticide in cases of illegitimacy, birth to the poor and old, and deformity, in the interest of bettering the State.

Descent in U.S. society, in contrast to the matriliny of the Navaho and the patriliny of the Chinese, is reckoned bilaterally: While the male family name is perpetuated, both parents (and their parents) are believed to contribute equally to descent groups. Reproduction in U.S. white middle-class society is generally not thought of as perpetuating long lines of descendants, but as building nuclear families, perhaps carrying on a family name; descent groups seldom include more than a few generations, and may do so through both males and females. Marriage is proscribed within these groups but is otherwise thought of as a matter of choice and free arrangement between the mates concerned. Occasionally choices are motivated by interests in building further "connections," but more often marriage is regarded as the consummation of an emotional commitment of love. Children also are thought of as the product and continuation of this commitment. Postmarital residence is generally not with the parents of either spouse, but in a separate dwelling.

It is difficult to discover from the social science literature the beliefs, values, and practices of middle-class whites regarding the menstrual cycle; it is perhaps assumed that "scientific" knowledge is widely dispersed in this group. Jordan (37) has shown that in a feminist clinic, women have an awareness of their pregnancy state which exceeds that available by medical diagnosis. Common use of various contraceptive techniques indicates great dispersion of knowledge; yet increasing rates of teenage pregnancy suggest that such knowledge is acquired later

(38, 39) (or that these pregnancies are wanted). There is evidence also (40, 41) that, at least among lower class women, beliefs about the menstrual cycle differ significantly from the scientific understanding; these women are reported to believe themselves fertile during and following menstruation but not otherwise. Newman (40) reports a belief among private clinic women that males and females are conceived at different points during the menstrual cycle. British women surveyed in an international study (42) (and presumably similar to U.S. white women in their reproductive beliefs) stand out from others surveyed (mostly Asian and Near Eastern) in several regards. They do not consider menstruation essential to femininity; they do not believe menses indicative of sickness or pollution; few regard menstruation as harmful to self or others; and only half avoid intercourse during menstruation.

The mother's behavior, activity, nutrition, and emotional state are thought to influence and to "mark" the fetus and child (40, 43). The fetus's activity level and position are believed indicative of its sex. Beliefs about diet, activity, and other restrictions are often adaptations from biomedical views (and vice versa). Birth, if not pregnancy, is regarded as an unclean (2) and a medical (if not a pathological) condition; this is evidenced by the fact that, at the turn of the twentieth century, 5 percent of births occurred in hospitals, whereas now only 5 percent occur out of hospitals (3, 44). Obstetricians rather than parturients are often said to "deliver" babies.

Until recently, white middle-class reproductive ideologies and perinatal ethics have differed along the lines of traditional religious denominations: Protestant, Catholic, and Jewish. Believing that contraception and abortion were human interferences in spiritual affairs, Catholics have been more prone to use rhythm, and far less prone to use other contraceptive methods (45). Protestants have sought smaller families, have used sterilization and other contraceptive methods (45), and have supported the morality of abortion at least under certain circumstances (46). Jews regard the fetus as part of the mother until birth and not as a separate human being (2). They have sought still smaller families, and have been yet more receptive to contraceptive methods (45) and abortion (46).

The legal status of the fetus is controversial and in contention. In half (24, 50) of the states the fetus is not regarded as a person, so that someone responsible for its uterine death, for example, in automobile injury, cannot be prosecuted for homicide (47). In contrast, several cases have recently appeared in which, on physicians' recommendations, the court has ordered cesarean delivery for the supposed protection of the fetus's well-being (48); the "rights" of the fetus are presumed to prevail over those of the mother, and the mother is assumed to be incompetent to judge or determine outcome. Similar legal action and controversy has accompanied efforts to sterilize patients judged incompetent in and outside of mental institutions (49, 50).

While views in the United States still differ along traditional religious lines, these differences have decreased (45). Another powerful division has recently gained strength—that between the worlds of "pro-life" and "pro-choice" proponents. Underlying this debate, at one level, is a difference in view of human beings, of males and females, their development, of responsibility, and of moral order and its bases. The two worlds and their histories are lucidly portrayed in Luker's *Abortion and the Politics of Motherhood*. Luker points out that

[T]he abortion debate is not about "facts" but about how to weigh, measure, and assess facts. . . . The two sides therefore examine exactly the same set of "facts" but come to diametrically opposed conclusions about them (35: p. 5).

Underlying the pro-life world view is firm belief in a divine moral order and plan. The divine plan is the source of moral principles, rewards, and sanctions; interference with this order and plan is regarded as extreme arrogance, morally wrong. In this plan, males and females are assigned distinctive, complementary natures and roles: Men work in the public world; women rear children and care for home and husband. Divinely ordered reproduction is seen as the essence of male-female relations, sanctioned by marriage; married couples are assumed to desire children, both as sacred duty and as pleasure. Nonmarital sex, indeed sexual relations precluding conception, are seen as blasphemous interference. Contraception (other than "natural family planning") and abortion are seen as morally wrong, as is family planning itself—the planning of the numbers and spacing of children. Since the fetus (and even the conceptus) is regarded as a human being, abortion and even intrauterine devices are seen as murder; judgments regarding "potential life" are seen as presumptuous. State and other institutional programs to assist parents and children are seen as an encroachment on an essential, sacred family function.

Underlying the pro-choice world view is a commitment to fulfilling the potential of individuals. This view may be grounded in religious conviction, but Luker claims that pro-choice advocates are pluralists who allow differing religions and moral schemes. The ideal of "procreational privacy" is one that has received support in the courts (49). Men and women are regarded as substantially equal. The development of individual autonomy and choice are emphasized for both. Sexual relations may be thought of as transcendent, not as fulfilling a sacred mandate, but rather as a means of unifying partners, of signaling unity, and of giving "one a sense of the infinite" (35: p. 178). The propriety of nonmarital sexual relations is also thought to be a matter of individual choice, based on the quality of interpersonal relations. For pro-choice adherents reproduction is also a matter of individual choice; though abortion is not undertaken lightly, both it and contraception are held to facilitate choice and the fulfillment of individual potential. The fetus is not thought of as a person until it is viable at birth; parents then regard their role as the provision of the best opportunities possible for the child's well-being and fulfilled potential (51). Reason, planning, and intervention are regarded as responsible rather than arrogant; lack of reproductive control is regarded as irresponsible in that children may be born unwanted and improperly cared for, and mothers may be harmed as well.

The introduction of new and experimental technologies of reproduction, obstetrics, and neonatology has significantly altered the ideology and relations involved in these issues. Viability of the fetus and newborn and the potential for the control of viability (for example, through genetic manipulation) have expanded radically. Indeed these changes call for extension of cultural understanding, value, and practice; this will not be easily achieved in a domain of radically opposed positions. As Annas (52) points out, while contraceptive discoveries made possible sex without reproduction, medicine has now made possible reproduction without sex, by *in vitro* fertilization, artificial insemination by donor, and surrogate embryo transfer. We will have to revise our concepts of parenthood and responsibility, the role and responsibility of medical and other practitioners, and the status and relations of the fetus and the newborn at various stages. The development of amniocentesis, fetal surgery, and fetal monitoring will also force reexamination of notions of community knowledge and the distribution of responsibility, accountability and self-determination. (See, for example, Rapp's [53] and Rivière's [54] discussion of the Warnock Report in Great Britain, which gives great weight to supposed genetic relations as "natural" and "God given.") The epidemic of malpractice suits indicates widespread misunderstanding about medical capacities and responsibilities.

The growth of neonatology and neonatal intensive care nurseries has given "new life" (54) to an issue with a long and diverse history (55, 56), otherwise thought of as abhorrent in contemporary Western society, namely infanticide. While a technology may enhance a certain outcome, the uncertainties of its early (if not later) use often create new damage as well. Since it may not be known who the technology may best serve, or the conditions for maximum efficacy, some patients may suffer more with the technology than they would have otherwise. The question here concerns the status of the severely disabled infant and the responsibility of others—parent, medical and other personnel, and society—in determining and controlling its future. Responses to the issue have generally followed along the divide between pro-life and pro-choice. The notorious case of "Baby Doe" has recently been "resolved" in a manner superficially satisfactory to both sides without significantly altering standard medical practice (57).

Lower Class Blacks

Lower class blacks are reported (41, 58; but see 59) to make a fairly clear-cut division between "natural" and "unnatural" sources of sickness and misfortune, and parallel sources of healing and redress. Natural problems arise from the natural environment, from improper (that is, opposing the Commandments) and immoderate behavior (thus the sufferer's responsibility), and from divine punishment. Religion is said to pervade black thinking about daily life and health. Unnatural problems arise from witchcraft and voodoo, the evil machinations of beings who work effects beyond the pale of nature, and unnatural events are sometimes ascribed to the devil (58). Physicians of Western medicine are thought to be capable with natural conditions, but ignorant of and ineffective (and even counterproductive) with unnatural conditions; here spiritualist healers are understanding and powerful, blessed with a Gift of God (41). The spirits of the deceased may be consulted; prayer and dreams, and vision are used in the diagnosis and treatment of problems (41). The assistance of physicians is sought for access to drugs, but not from respect for their superior knowledge. Black beliefs described by Snow combine theological and spiritist, astrological, humoral, and sympathetic magic traditions with versions of "scientific" medicine. Perhaps akin to the "epistemological modesty" ascribed to the Chinese by Unschuld (35), Snow notes a broad acceptance of different ideas in her informants:

Informants rarely categorically denied anything. A statement might be made that they did not believe in something, witchcraft, say, or marking children. Almost always they would go on to say that it might be POSSIBLE, but they had not experienced it (41: pp. 33–34).

Stack (60) argues that common notions of "nuclear family" and "household" hinder an understanding of lower class black social life. Patterns of interaction (or eating, sleeping, sharing, and exchange) are shaped by "personal kindreds"; kindreds are created from both (genealogical) kinsmen and "fictive" kin. Snow (41) reports that more than half of the households in her study were headed by women; 17 percent were headed by men, the remainder (33 percent) by couples. Gabriel and McAnarney (61) report that for young black women, pregnancy and childbirth initiate the transition to adulthood; motherhood does not require prior education, marriage, or independent living arrangements, and young pregnancy is often neither "unwanted" nor "illegitimate." (One-fourth of births among blacks are to women younger than 20 years.) Premarital sex is widely accepted (41). Relations with males during this period are described as "tenuous," and the young mother's own family provides support. "Fathers' may be actively involved as social parents, but they may also withdraw from this relationship. Their chosen participation establishes and validates their parental rights.

Although Blacks acquire kin through their mothers and fathers, the economic insecurity of the black male, and the availability of welfare to the female-child unit, makes it difficult for an unemployed Black husband-father to compete with a woman's kin for authority and for control over her children (60: pp. 117–18).

Infants born in these circumstances are often adopted by their grandmothers who then raise them and become their "mothers."

Blood figures prominently in black notions of pathology; the body is thought to be dirty (41), and healing is often thought to require the rebalance of blood whose qualities have gone to extremes. This complex may be associated with the constitutional weakness attributed to women. Women are regarded as particularly susceptible to pathology at times of menstruation, abortion, and childbirth. Menstruation is thought of as the body's means of expelling dirty blood. Interference with this cleansing, for example by contraceptive methods that change blood flow, is avoided (58,61). Sex is also avoided around the menstrual period in order to preclude contamination. It is also believed that the uterus is closed between menses, thus preventing the invasion of both pathogenic forces and agents and semen, and thus conception. Sexual potency is seen not only as a procreative power but as an index of general health; babies, children, and postmenopausal women are felt to have weaker bodies (41).

The fetus is regarded as highly susceptible to influence by the mother's behavior. It will be "marked," deformed or disabled, if the mother behaves immoderately, for example, laughing at a crippled person (40, 58). Fetuses are also subject to the evil thoughts and curses of others. Their health thus depends on mutual and responsible social behavior. Snow (41) claims that several "magical" practices are associated with the enhancement and control of bleeding, pregnancy, and birth. Labor pains are thought of as divine punishment.

Childbearing is said to be "natural" and highly desirable (60). Yet, while no norms regarding infanticide are reported, it should be noted that vital statistics, perhaps biased, indicate a rate of homicide in black infants (less than one year of age) three times that found among whites, though a smaller ratio than found for other age categories (62). Children are thought to require strict guidance in proper living. Punishment and spanking are thought to be good for body and soul (41).

The Perinatal World View of Obstetrics and Biomedicine

While it would be as prejudicial to claim that "All obstetricians (or all physicians) believe . . ." as to claim that "All Navaho believe . . ." or "All Chinese believe . . . ," we may nevertheless ascribe cultural tendencies of belief, value, and practice to obstetricians and other medical specialists (43, 63, 64). By an examination of textual material and technical and other practices, we may interpret underlying notions of agents, their capacities, and their development, of causality and responsibility, rights, and ethics. In the same way that wide diversity is found on perinatal ethics within American populations generally, similar diversity may be found among professional birth attendants. (As Arney [43] notes, there are also several opposed interpretations of obstetrical practice and its history: those of the profession justifying its practice, those of feminist critics finding and resisting domination, those of governmental agencies creating and enforcing law, and allocating resources for research, technology, and medical care, and those of historians, professing to have no axes to grind.)

A useful window into the world of obstetrics is provided by a review of the current and recent editions of *Williams Obstetrics* (65), the standard textbook in the field. Changes in *Williams* reflect changes within the specialty as well as its responses to social and political change beyond. Remarkable, for example, are altered conceptions of participants in and around the profession, of their status, of patients and their consociates, of the patients' status and control of their courses, of what is available and provided for them, and of the role ascribed to nonmedical disciplines.

The fifteenth edition (66) continues and expands an introductory chapter, "Obstetrics in Broad Perspective," including the sweeping principle that, "In a broader sense, obstetrics is concerned with reproduction of a society." The relevance of nonmedical disciplines—psychology, sociology, economics, nutrition, and the law—is proclaimed, though not pursued in any detail. A chapter on "Psychosomatic Aspects of Obstetrics" found in the thirteenth edition (67) is deleted in all later editions. The notion of obstetrician as analgesic is asserted, and the sources of this power ascribed to clinical experience rather than to scientific principles and deliberate instruction.

[H]e must instill in her not only confidence but also the feeling that he is her medically wise friend, sincerely desirous of sparing her all possible pain within the limit of safety for her and her child. The very process of such a doctor is in itself a potent analgesic. These qualities, however, are not easily organized into a code of instructions, but result only from the experience of long nights in the labor room coupled with understanding and sympathy. They are at once the essence of good clinical medicine and the safest and most welcome of obstetric anodynes (67: p. 410).

Another chapter titled "Maternal Physiology in Pregnancy" in the fourteenth edition (68) is seemingly broadened to "Maternal Adaptation to Pregnancy" in the fifteenth (66); yet the adaptation considered is strictly physiological; that is, even within the "Broad Perspective," maternal adaptation is not thought to include the woman's experience (6).

Women and other participants come to be included as attendants. While the thirteenth edition (67) is dedicated to "residents and their wives," and the fourteenth (68) to "men of purpose," the fifteenth (66) is dedicated to "physicians, nurses, and many others" concerned with obstetrical issues; the sixteenth (69) is personally dedicated to two named women, presumably the wives of two of the authors. (An index entry referring to all pages in each volume, "Chauvinism, male, variable amounts," appears in the fifteenth [66], expands to "voluminous amounts" in the sixteenth [69], and is expunged in the seventeenth [65].)

Recent editions of *Williams* note increasingly the problem of world population growth, and the need for family planning services, including contraception. The position adopted here is practially that of pro-choice proponents. Physicians are advised to be knowledgeable and to provide contraception despite possible variations in their own beliefs.

Obstetricians will vary in their attitudes toward contraception, but they cannot avoid their responsibility since the health of the mother and her family are dependent on the spacing and limitation of her children (68: p. 1099).

Women who wish not to become pregnant, *Williams* recommends, should be given contraceptives, no matter how young. (No suggestion is either made or not made regarding parental awareness or consent; deliberate or not, this omission seems to empower the individual patient of any age.)

In the fourteenth edition (68) two forms of induced abortions are recognized: therapeutic and illegal. In the fifteenth edition (66) (following *Roe v. Wade*, 1973), elective abortions are further distinguished— chosen not for the mother's health (physiologically defined), but for some "subjective" reason of her own. In considering the justification for contraception and abortion, *Williams* insists on the importance and responsibility of postnatal care as well as prenatal care.

If a child is to be born, means for providing appropriate care for that child BEFORE AND AFTER birth must be readily available. . . . Unfortunately, strong opponents of abortion, all too frequently, have also opposed the dissemination and application of effective contraceptive techniques (66: p. 478).

Increasingly in recent editions of *Williams* (since the fourteenth edition), most births are said to be normal, physiological processes, and not pathological.

A priori pregnancy should be considered a normal physiologic state. Unfortunately, the complexity of the functional and anatomic changes that accompany gestation tend in the minds of some to stigmatize normal pregnancy as a disease process (68: p. 245).

Reassurance of the parturient that this is so is thought to alleviate some of her anxiety and to reduce her pain. Yet this proclamation does not appear to be consistent with either the vast detailing of pathology in the rest of the text or the routinized apparatus and technical procedures followed for even "normal" births in medical settings otherwise concerned with pathology. Moreover, the chapter in *Williams* on normal birth also equates "physiologic birth" with so-called natural childbirth; obstetricians are advised to assist their patients who may wish to follow this "school of thought," one distinct from the normal birth procedures they recommend. Thus a birth described as "normal" and "physiologic" is set apart from one that is "natural" and also "physiologic." Normal birth is medical, if not pathological.

Notions of the obstetric patient have expanded radically. While the development of fetal medicine is noted in preceding editions, this specialty is given a new and separate chapter in the fifteenth edition (66). The following edition (69) describes the fetus as the "second patient," and the current (seventeenth) edition asserts the fetus's "many rights and privileges, comparable to those previously achieved only after birth" (65: p. xi). The status of the fetus as rightful, privileged patient raises a host of issues noted earlier.

Arney (43) cites the sixteenth edition of the introduction, "Obstetrics in Broad Perspective," in his own preface, without comment, but presumably as an indication of the acknowledgment by obstetricians of psychological and social issues surrounding and directly relevant to events of birth. Arney argues that since 1945, the profession of obstetrics has maintained its authority and power by adopting an ecological view of childbirth, to include psychological and social aspects, to collaborate with a "team" of attendants, to respond to the concerns of parturient women, and to address the issues raised by ethicists. Arney does not remark, however, on the gulf which separates the six pages of the introductory chapter of *Williams* from the rest of the book. The remainder of the book makes almost no mention of the physiological and social issues noted at the outset to affect profoundly the quantitative and qualitative aspects of human reproduction. The substance of the book reviews obstetrics in the "traditional" manner, narrowly, according to its own introductory comments. If these issues are as important in a broad perspective as physiological ones, why is there not one chapter about them? Arney mistakes express intention for its fulfillment, and text for practice.

On the other hand, Arney usefully portrays several epistemological and metaphysical principles underlying the world view of obstetrics. He reviews the literature on fetal monitoring and finds little evidence to favor its routine use; yet fetal monitoring is used routinely and justified on supposedly scientific grounds. Arney refers to this partial, selective use of available evidence as "scientistic" (in contrast to a more rational, "scientific" evaluation): science is a standard professed to justify practices, but it is not followed. The availability of a technology with claimed effect seems to compel use to this end, despite inadequate evidence (see also 70).

Arney also shows that ethical decisions within the profession are represented, at least to outsiders, as based not on judgment, but on rational clinical grounds. Similar ideologies are found in medicine more broadly; science may be thought to logically dictate choice, thus supposedly avoiding subjective judgment (71).

Conclusion

A brief excursion through five cultural settings indicates radical differences in worlds perceived and, perhaps to a lesser extent, worlds inhabited. These reports from near and far may be erroneous in some details; but, if we do not suffer from some large and widespread anthropological illusion, large differences exist among human cultures. The fact of these differences, and some of the specific differences themselves, carry profound implications for the development of an ethical theory, of ethical principles, and, more relevant here, of perinatal ethics.

1. Human nature is far more varied than Westerners (including philosophers) are accustomed to acknowledge. The identities and qualities of beings in the world, their development, their achievement and loss of capacities, their relations with one another, and ideologies of purpose and its justification differ systematically from society to society. Such variation, moreover, may exist not only between cultural groups, but within them; indeed cultural and ethical conflicts may rage within individuals. An ethical theory and ethical principles are rooted in just such notions—of what kinds of beings there are, their capacities, and so on.

2. A troublesome, but vital epistemological issue arises here. Given the great diversity in world views, is there some reasonable vantage from which to examine the validity or the relative worth of these systems, or to judge even parts of them? Can we determine conclusively, for example, whether human life begins at conception? Or, assuming for the moment that is does begin at conception, whether or under what conditions the manipulation or the "killing" of this new being would be immoral? It seems unlikely that an omniscient, entirely value-neutral vantage could be established on some culturally unbiased, "purely logical," grounds.

3. It seems less likely still that adherents to these diverse positions would accept such a culturally neutral position (assuming it could be made comprehensible to them), or that they would even embrace either the principles or the "facts" on which it was based. Such historically and culturally rooted positions, moreover, are often not held lightly, but pursued with undying passion.

4. Given this essential pluralism and the limits of abstract, impersonal, and culture-free reason, three major alternative responses for the development of a perinatal ethics seem possible:

a) Ethical anarchy, in which each system is left on its own to achieve its ends by its chosen means. This nonchoice position would seem to foster perpetual misunderstanding, if not relentless warfare, since the goals and means of one group might violate the essential beliefs of another group unconscionably, thus perhaps calling for repressive response.

b) Ethical absolutism, in which warfare is carried out; one system, however derived and formulated, is imposed and required for everyone, and alternatives are eliminated. (Such a "solution" would have to justify its own domination and the elimination of alternatives.)

c) An ethics and public policy of compromise and consensus in which no absolute ethical standard from any one position is imposed on anyone, but choice among alternatives is maximized insofar as its does not compromise the choices of others. (This position may be regarded as itself a compromise between absolutism and anarchy.) Achievement of such a position is at once necessary and impossible: necessary because cultural plurality is an essential facet of human nature, and because an ethics must be based on an understanding of human function and purpose; impossible because an ethics *without some* overriding standards would be meaningless, while an ethics *with some* overriding standards is likely to approximate the standards of some groups and to violate those of other groups. Compromise and consensus will be regarded as a failure by the proponents of any system which includes certain inviolable absolutes. Pluralistic choice among various alternatives may be regarded as sacrilegious arrogance by some and as a societal ideal by others.

An ethics of compromise and consensus would, for example, seem to favor the pro-choice position insofar as it allowed for alternatives rather than insisting on a single correct position. Yet this inclination would lead only to a partial and somewhat arbitrary solution. A compromise ethics would still have to demarcate a borderline between legitimate and immoral killings of conceptus, fetus, and infant. And while such a decision might refer to scientific knowledge and established technical procedures, these would by no means dictate an ethical choice. Such choices will have to be made by consensus which will inevitably require mutual concessions and less than total certainty that one's own view is the only tolerable one.

Ethical theories and principles which are not at least implicitly anthropological—addressing world views, values, and practices other than those of their proponents—are culture-bound, parochial, presumptuous. Many controversies in perinatal ethics involve differences which cannot be eliminated by abstract, culture-neutral reason. They involve conflicts among understandings, values, and practices that are rooted in particular historical settings. An anthropological perspective is basic to an adequate account of the nature and depth of such conflicts. It insists on the importance of history and society and on communication across these boundaries. Toward the resolution of conflicts an anthropological perspective fosters mutual understanding but does not invite easy answers or simple prescriptions.

References

1. Ford CS. A comparative study of human reproduction. New Haven CT: Yale U Publications in Anthropology 32, 1945.
2. Mead M, Newton N. Cultural patterning of perinatal behavior. In: Richardson SA, Guttmacher AF, eds, Childbearing—its social and psychological aspects. Baltimore: Williams and Wilkins, 1967.

3. Jordan B. Birth in four cultures. Montreal: Eden Press, 1983.
4. Kay MA. The anthropology of human birth, Philadelphia: FA Davis, 1982.
5. Faithorn E. The concept of pollution among the Kafe of the Papua New Guinea Highlands. In: Reiter RR, ed, Toward an anthropology of women. New York: Monthly Review Press, 1975.
6. Young IM. Pregnant embodiment: subjectivity and alienation. J Med Philos 1984;9:45–62.
7. Leach ER. Virgin birth. Proc Roy Anthrop Inst 1967;39–50.
8. Firth R. Twins, birds, and vegetables: problems of identification in primitive religious thought. Man 1966;1:1–17.
9. Devereux G. A study of abortion in primitive society. New York: International Universities Press. 1976 (originally 1955).
10. Hahn RA. Understanding beliefs: an essay on the methodology of the statement and analysis of belief systems. Current Anthropol 1973;14:207–209.
11. Korbin J, ed. Child abuse and neglect: cross-cultural perspectives. Berkeley: U of California Press, 1981.
12. Witherspoon G. Language and art in the Navajo universe. Ann Arbor: U of Michigan Press, 1977.
13. Kunitz SJ, Levy JE. Navajos. In: Harwood A, ed, Ethnicity and medical care. Cambridge MA: Harvard U Press, 1981.
14. Ladd J. The structure of a moral code: a philosophical analysis of ethical discourse applied to the ethics of the Navaho Indians. Cambridge MA: Harvard U Press, 1957.
15. Levy JE. Traditional Navajo health beliefs and practices. In: Kunitz SJ, ed, Disease and the role of medicine: the Navajo experience. Berkeley: U of California Press, 1983.
16. Lamphere L. Strategies, cooperation, and conflict among women's domestic groups. In: Rosaldo M, Lamphere L, eds, Women, culture and society. Palo Alto CA: Stanford U Press. 1974.
17. Bailey F. Some sex beliefs and practices in a Navajo community. Papers of the Peabody Museum of American Archeology and Ethnology 1950;40:2.
18. Frisbie C. Kinaalda: a study of the Navajo girl's puberty ceremony. Middletown CT: Wesleyan U Press, 1967.
19. Wright A. Attitudes toward childbearing and menstruation among the Navajo. In: Kay MA, ed, The anthropology of human birth. Philadelphia: FA Davis, 1982.
20. Newton N, Newton M. Childbirth in crosscultural perspective. In: Howells JG, ed, Modern perspectives in psycho-obstetrics. Edinburgh: Oliver and Boyd, 1972.
21. Hahn RA. Culture and informed consent: an anthropological perspective. President's Commission for the Study of Ethical Problems in Medicine and Biomedical and Behavioral Research, Making Healthcare Decisions, Volume 3, Appendices Studies on the Foundations of Informed Consent. Washington DC: 1982.
22. Fox RC, Swazey JP. Medical morality is not bioethics—medical ethics in China and the United States. Persp Biol Med 1984;27(3)336–60.
23. Farquhar J. Time and text: approaching contemporary Chinese medical practice through analysis of a published case. Paper presented at the Annual Meetings of the American Anthropological Association, Washington, DC, Dec 1985.

24. Porkert M. The theoretical foundations of Chinese medicine. Cambridge MA: MIT Press, 1974.
25. Unschuld P. Epistemological issues and changing legitimation. Traditional Chinese medicine in the 20th century. Paper presented at the Annual Meetings of the American Anthropological Association, Washington DC, Dec 1985.
26. Pillsbury BLK. 'Doing the month': confinement and convalescence of Chinese women after childbirth. In: Kay MA, ed, The anthropology of human birth. Philadelphia: FA Davis, 1982.
27. Char EL. The Chinese American. In: Clark AL, ed, Culture and childrearing. Philadelphia: FA Davis, 1981.
28. Fawcett JT, Arnold F, Bulatao RA, et al. The value of children in Asia and the United States: comparative perspectives. Papers of the East-West Population Institute 1974;32.
29. Kleinman AM. Patients and healers in the context of culture. Berkeley: U of California Press, 1980.
30. Johnson EL. Women and childbearing in Kwan Mun Hau village: a study of social change. In: Wolf M, Witke R, eds, Women in Chinese society. Palo Alto CA: Stanford U Press, 1975.
31. Ahearn EM. The power and pollution of Chinese women. In: Wolf M, Witke R, eds, Women in Chinese society. Palo Alto CA: Stanford U Press, 1975.
32. Topley M. Cosmic antagonisms: a mother-child syndrome. In: Wolfe A, ed, Religious ritual in Chinese society. Palo Alto CA: Stanford U Press, 1974.
33. Rose PA. The Chinese American. In: Clark AL, ed, Culture, childbearing, health professionals. Philadelphia: FA Davis, 1978.
34. Hahn, RA. Rethinking 'disease' and 'illness'. In: Daniel EV, Pugh J eds, South Asian systems of healing. Contrib Asian Studies 1984;18:1–23.
35. Luker K. Abortion and the politics of motherhood. Berkeley: U California Press, 1984.
36. Carrick P. Medical ethics in antiquity. Boston: D Reidel, 1985.
37. Jordan B. The self-diagnosis of early pregnancy: an investigation of lay competence. Medical Anthropol 1977;1(2):1.
38. Kisker EE. Teenagers talk about sex, pregnancy and contraception. Family Planning Persp 1985;17(2):83–91.
39. Morrison D. Adolescent contraceptive behavior: a review. Psych Bull 1985;98(3):538–68.
40. Newman LF. Folklore of pregnancy: wives' tales in Contra Costa County, California. Western Folklore 1969;28(2):112–35.
41. Snow L. Popular medicine in a black neighborhood. In Spicer EH, ed, Ethnic medicine in the Southwest. Tucson: University of Arizona Press, 1977.
42. W.H.O. Task Force on Psychosocial Research in Family Planning, Special Programme of Research, Development and Research Training in Human Reproduction. A cross-cultural study of menstruation: implications for contraceptive development and use. Studies in Family Planning. 1981;12(1):3–16.
43. Arney WR. Power and the profession of obstetrics. Chicago: U of Chicago Press, 1982.

44. Wertz RW, Wertz DC. Lying-in: a history of childbirth in America. New York: Schocken, 1979 (1977).
45. Mosher WD, Goldscheider C. Contraceptive patterns of religious and racial groups in the United States, 1955–76: convergence and distinctiveness. Studies in Family Planning 1984;15(3):101–11.
46. Forrest JD, Henshaw SK. What U.S. women think and do about contraception. Family Planning Persp 1983;15(4):157–66.
47. Washington Post, Minnesota's high court rules fetus is not a human being. Dec 7, 1985.
48. Irwin S, Jordan B. Court-ordered cesarean sections: an anthropological perspective. Paper presented at Annual Meetings of the American Anthropological Association, Washington DC, Dec 1985.
49. Friedman JM. Sterilization: legal aspects. Encyclopedia of Bioethics. New York: Free Press. 1978.
50. Petchesky RP. Reproduction, ethics, and public policy: the federal sterilization regulations. Hastings Cent Rep 1979;29–41.
51. Fischer JL, Fischer A. The New Englanders of Orchard Town, U.S.A. New York: John Wiley, 1966.
52. Annas GJ. Redefining parenthood and protecting embryos: why we need new laws. Hastings Cent Rep 1984:50–52.
53. Rapp R. Moral pioneers: women, men and fetuses on a frontier of reproductive technology. Paper presented at Annual Meetings of the American Anthropological Association. Washington, DC, Dec 1985.
54. Rivière P. Unscrambling parenthood: the Warnock report. Anthropol Today 1985;1(4):2–7.
55. Williamson L. Infanticide: an anthropological analysis. In: Kohl M, ed, Infanticide and the value of life. Buffalo: Prometheus Books, 1978.
56. Tooley M. Abortion and infanticide. Oxford: Clarendon Press, 1983.
57. Murray TH. The final, anticlimactic rule of Baby Doe. Hastings Cent Rep 1985:5–9.
58. Snow LF. Traditional health beliefs and practices among lower class black Americans. Western J Med 1983;139:820–28.
59. Jackson JJ. Urban black Americans. In: Harwood A, ed, Ethnicity and medical care. Cambridge MA: Harvard U Press, 1981.
60. Stack CB. All our kin. New York: Harper Collophon, 1974.
61. Gabriel A, McAnarney ER. Parenthood in two subcultures: white, middleclass couples and black, low-income adolescents in Rochester, New York. Adolescence 1983;18(71):595–608.
62. U.S. Department of Health and Human Services. Health United States 1984. Hyattsville MD: U.S. Public Health Service, 1984.
63. Hahn RA, Gaines AD. Physicians of Western medicine. Dordrecht, Holland: D Reidel, 1985.
64. Lock M. Models and practice in medicine: menopause as syndrome or life transition? In: Hahn RA, Gaines AD, eds, Physicians of Western medicine. Dordrecht, Holland: D Reidel, 1985.
65. Pritchard JA, MacDonald PC, Gant NF. Williams obstetrics, 17th ed. New York: Appleton-Century-Crofts, 1985.
66. Pritchard JA, Macdonald PC. Williams obstetrics, 15th ed. New York: Appleton-Century-Crofts, 1976.

67. Eastman NJ, Hellman LM. Williams obstetrics, 13th ed. New York: Appleton-Century-Crofts, 1966.
68. Hellman LM, Pritchard JA. Williams obstetrics, 14th ed. New York: Appleton-Century-Crofts, 1971.
69. Pritchard JA, Macdonald PC. Williams obstetrics, 16th ed. New York: Appleton-Century-Crofts, 1981.
70. Marieskind H. Women in the health system: Patients, providers, and programs. St. Louis: CV Mosby, 1980.
71. Hahn RA. A world of internal medicine; Portrait of an internist. In: Hahn RA, Gaines AD, eds, Physicians of Western medicine. Dordrecht, Holland: D Reidel, 1985.

9

So Maybe It's Wrong: Should We *Do* Anything about It? Ethics and Social Policy

THOMAS H. MURRAY

Deciding the morality of a host of practices at the outset of life is difficult enough. An entirely new set of ethical questions arises once we ask what society should do in response. For example, if we judge that some things like surrogate pregnancies are morally wrong, what if anything should we do to discourage them? Should we imprison the women who bear surrogate children or sterilize them? Should we imprison the parents who commissioned the surrogate pregnancy or ban them from future adoptions? Should we disbar the attorneys who arrange the contracts? Or, as we are doing in most states, should we simply refuse to enforce the contracts (and possibly, threaten the parties with prosecution under the state statute banning the sale of children) (1)?

The first several options appear much too Draconian for our taste, meaning simply that these responses seem out of proportion to the wrong they seek to discourage. They may be either too severe a punishment or carry in their train such damaging consequences that, even if not unjust, they are unwise. Policymakers rarely (I do not say *never*) propose such outrageous options. What that shows, I think, is that we accept that social policy responses to practices we disapprove of morally must themselves be morally acceptable. You do not kill a mosquito with a sledgehammer because that would be a disproportionate response to the threat and because you might damage the more valuable furniture on which the mosquito has alighted.

Societies are responsible for setting public policies to encourage, permit, or discourage practices at the outset of life. It is always possible to think of the moral dimensions of social policies. But there are nonmoral values typically at stake as well when policies must be considered. Efficiency, though sometimes falsely enshrined by economists as the only important value, is nonetheless a significant nonmoral value that ought to be weighed, along with other values, in fashioning policies. Even if we limit ourselves to moral values, there will be several that become relevant at the level of policy that were not relevant to the judgment whether a particular act or practice was ethically justifiable.

This might seem contradictory, but an example should prove otherwise. Many of us might be convinced that abortion is the wrongful taking of human life. On that ground alone, we could feel justified in trying to ban abortions, and perhaps even have it included in criminal statutes as murder, so that physicians performing abortions could be prosecuted for homicide, women procuring abortions prosecuted for conspiracy to commit homicide, nurses as accessories to homicide, and so on. All these things would be consistent with our deep convictions about the profound immorality of abortion. But we live in a culture where most people do not share our beliefs. To the majority, most early abortions, while not acts of moral indifference, are much less than the murder of a person. And the majority favors permitting abortions, even though they are uneasy about some of them.

What would happen if the convinced minority succeeded in imposing its will on the majority? Those individuals would have achieved their goal of discouraging officially a practice they believe is seriously immoral, and in that way they will have met their obligation to do what they believe is right. But by imposing their will on so many others, they will have threatened other moral values, perhaps equally dear. They will force others to pursue their vision of human good furtively. In all likelihood, abortions will continue to be done, though under more dangerous conditions; therefore, some women will be injured or killed. A number of good people will commit what will now be defined as criminal acts. Widespread disobedience to the law and resentment against what will be seen as the imposition of oppressive and unjustified rules will feed discontent and loosen the bonds of social solidarity. Disobedience of one law may lead to disrespect for the law in general. The price, then, of a social policy intended to bolster one moral value may be terribly high: nothing less than an attrition of other moral values, values crucial to sustaining the social fabric.

What I want to do in this chapter is give some sense of the kinds of values that come into play at the level of social policy, and to stress the independent importance of them over and above the values determining the morality of the particular practice, be it abortion, IVF, or decision making for seriously ill newborns. If we choose to encourage or discourage something, the possible ways of doing so are not much limited by human imagination: we can think of many more means than we would ever consider employing. They will vary in several nonmoral respects, including political feasibility, practicality, and efficiency. They will also vary in moral respects: Is a particular method just in its allocation of resources and in its distribution of burdens and benefits? Is it unduly coercive? Does it diminish liberty or privacy? Any or all of these considerations may be relevant to the ethics of a proposed social policy, and hence, to the question of social responsibility.

It would be a mistake to think that the only kinds of social policies with moral relevance are those aimed at stopping an unwanted activity. I will call these *negative* policies since their direct intended impact is to prevent something. Of course, negative policies will always have positive goals as well. Prohibition's goals included reducing crime and social disorganization thought to be the result of alcohol, and promoting health. It would make little sense to force people to stop drinking unless there were some sought-after positive social consequences that were presumed to follow. But, since the direct, declared impact of the policy was to discourage rather than promote an activity (in this instance, by making it illegal) it seems fair to call it a negative policy. In contrast, policies I will call *positive* are those explicitly designed to encourage a practice. For example, federal funding of research on *in vitro* fertilization would be a positive policy, aimed at promoting the perfection of this technique. The distinction between positive and negative policies is a fairly rough-and-ready one; not all policies will fit neatly into one or the other category. But it alerts us to the fact that social policies can promote as well as prohibit, and that the decision not to promote, by for example refusing to pay for IVF with public funds or insurance, is as much a social policy decision as a choice to ban it.

Distributive justice comes into play at the policy level. The contemporary United States has a double problem dealing with disputes over distributive justice. First is the need to adjudicate among competing claims: who is most deserving? But we do not even have broad social agreement about what makes one person more deserving than another. This is our second problem—competing theories about what justice consists of. Should we distribute according to need, according to social worth, or according to contribution? Yet in the face of both kinds of uncertainty and disagreement, we must still choose. "Permitting" a practice may be an empty liberty or a socially iniquitous injustice if only the wealthy benefit or only the poor are tempted to take advantage of it.

Another set of issues that arise when we consider policies are those where additional values become relevant. Suppose that we want to ban birth control (as did the state of Connecticut in the early 1960s). Even granting the contentious point that such a ban would be desirable, accomplishing it in practice necessarily brings in other important social values. How would the state enforce such a ban? Would it require "allow[ing] the police to search the sacred precincts of marital bedrooms for telltale signs of the use of contraceptives?" as the U.S. Supreme Court decision in *Griswold v. State of Connecticut* worried (2)? Even if we were convinced that the value sought by the policy were a sound one, we might still conclude that some approaches, at least, were so costly to other important values, in this case privacy, that they were, on balance, unwise. The other values impinged upon by a policy must be examined. The impulse to say, once we find something of which we disapprove, that "there ought to be a law against it," is one that often needs to be restrained.

A final point about social policies in general is that they usually have a number of significant *unintended* consequences along with the intended ones. These unintended consequences may be socially desirable or undesirable (as, for that matter, may be the intended consequences, although presumably the policy would not have been pursued had people intended and anticipated that negative consequences would predominate).

At this juncture, an example would be helpful. Take the matter of pregnancies among adolescents. Suppose a policy were enacted to provide intensive education on how to avoid pregnancy, and to supply effective contraceptives to adolescents. The primary intention is to avoid pregnancies among adolescents. Behind this undoubtedly lie several positive social goals, two of which are most likely to be intended: enhancing the life-chances of adolescent girls, for whom pregnancy often means the end of education and poorer prospects for employment, and lowering the number of babies born into the unfavorable circumstances of a poor, single-parent household.

Several other impacts are likely as well, including decreasing the number of very premature infants born in this country (adolescent mothers being more likely to give birth to small infants) which would result in lowering the neonatal and infant mortality rates (the incidence of premature, low-birthweight infants being the best predictor of these rates), and probably also resulting in lowered costs for neonatal intensive care and long-term care for the mentally and physically disabled. (Roughly half the admissions to NICUs are low birthweight infants. When they do not die quickly, they often require the most expensive and prolonged care. And, they are more likely than term infants to have long-term disabilities (3). Undesirable possible consequences include an increase in adolescent sexuality (viewed negatively by many, though not all people), the possible increase of sexually transmitted diseases among adolescents, and the further separation of sex from intimacy and commitment.

We could go even further and point out that an obviously good consequence—lowering the number of infants born prematurely—has some undesirable effects as well, such as lowering the demand for nurses and physicians in NICUs. Yet most of us would have no trouble saying that the good outweighs the bad in this particular trade-off. The general point is that social policies typically have a multitude of consequences, a mixture of intended and unintended, desirable and undesirable. These consequences will vary in several important respects: how probable they are; how powerful their impact; how strong the social consensus as to whether they are desirable or not, to name a few. Judging which policies to adopt requires considerable imagination to identify which consequences are likely to occur in significant measure, and a good deal of practical wisdom to weigh probability, importance, and social acceptability.

It would be difficult enough to do all this in a society where there was extensive agreement about the fundamentals of the social contract and about matters of everyday morality. But when the nation embraces a broad plurality of political and moral beliefs, as in the contemporary United States, the additional requirement arises to preserve, as far as possible, the neutrality of the state with respect to specific moral beliefs without at the same time sacrificing fundamental principles. To a considerable extent, then, social policy in a pluralistic state must concern itself with healing or at least not aggravating the splits in the body politic. In consequence, much of the pragmatics of policymaking are attempts to avoid social disruption. Many of the issues discussed in this book have the potential to be wedges, driving groups farther apart. Attending to this need to minimize divisiveness will help us understand better the dynamics of social policymaking.

Avoiding Divisive Social Policies

Preserving the peace may require a society to avoid taking sides in a dispute where fundamental values, firmly held, are in stark conflict. Probably no controversy more fully represents this sort of situation than abortion in the United States today. This is not simply an intellectual dispute over when protectable human life begins, over the moral relevance of potentiality, or over the privacy rights a woman holds with regard to her own body. Nor is it even simply a matter of the stark conflict between those who hold that abortion is nothing less than the murder of an innocent baby versus those who believe that it is, at least sometimes, much less than that, and less morally grave than a woman's interest in managing the circumstances of her life. This would be enough of a conflict. But Kristin Luker's book, *Abortion and the Politics of Motherhood*, shows that the value conflicts cut even deeper, into our core beliefs about the value women have in our culture, the roles that lend them dignity and purpose, the place of sexuality in human relationships, and the relative importance of chance and control in our lives (4).

Certainly, a society could adopt a policy that came down on one or the other side of this chasm. But even if the side chosen were that favored by a slim, or for that matter a considerable, majority, there would be great costs to peace and civility, as well as the sadness of loss accompanying an explicit, socially ordained renunciation of the most highly cherished values of many citizens. Whenever possible, a prudent society avoids such a choice. I believe it is plausible to think that this is the course generally followed in the abortion controversy—a refusal to fully uphold or renounce either side's values. On one level this is a political compromise, with the interests of both sides being given significant weight. But, in the instance of abortion, this is also a decision not to take sides in the moral debate. So, our laws neither give women complete control over the decision whether to continue a pregnancy, nor do they grant the full moral and legal status of personhood to the fetus. This strategy could be characterized as cowardly, but it would also be seen as a judicious effort to avoid the social costs of taking sides when the stakes are so dear.

Few people have been able to avoid thinking about abortion as a moral and political issue. Yet there are many other difficult questions, perhaps as potentially wrenching as abortion, but where there has not as yet been the same sort of profound and widespread polarization. Societies have a strong interest in managing questions like this so that their potential for social disruption is minimized. At least five problems at the outset of life may fit into this category: the moral status of an embryo *in vitro*; amniocentesis and the so-called hard reasons for abortion; the value of disabled persons; quality-of-life judgments; and whose interests should count in decision making for children.

What are our social responsibilities with respect to an issue such as the moral status of an in vitro embryo? While the "Human Life Amendment" to the U.S. Constitution was not directed primarily at IVF, it is nevertheless relevant, and it exemplifies one approach to such a controversy—pass a law enforcing a particular point of view (5). (Under a Constitutional amendment asserting that the newly fertilized ovum is a person for the purposes of law, would discarding several poorly developing embryos from a petri dish be multiple homicide?) Another approach is the one taken by Great Britain, which established the "Committee of Inquiry into Human Fertilisation and Embryology," better known as the Warnock Committee, which made no less than 64 specific recommendations, many of them for legislation (6). The Committee, however, tried very hard to avoid embracing any narrow point of view, which led predictably to accusations that they were inconsistent.

For example, the Warnock Committee recommended that *in vitro* fertilized embryos up to the end of the fourteenth day of development be permitted to be used in research. They even recommend allowing the *in vitro* production of human embryos specifically intended to be research materials. Yet at the same time they urge that "The embryo of the human species should be afforded some protection in law," that researchers should be licensed, and that "Any unauthorised use of an *in vitro* embryo would in itself constitute a criminal offence," as would any research use of an embryo older than 14 days' development (7).

What theory of the moral status of human embryos would embrace, without contradiction, all of these recommendations? It may be possible to find such a theory, though it is doubtful that the Committee's acceptance of 14 days as the watershed suffices. But the Committee did not need to provide a final, authoritative answer to this question. Its task was to find a compromise that would permit important social needs to be fulfilled, without outraging widely and deeply held moral values. The Committee did not argue that after 14 days a human embryo is, morally speaking, a full person; rather it said that before 14 days the case for embryonic personhood is weak (in that the cells have not even begun to differentiate into those that will become the fetus and those that will become the placenta, cord, and so on). Since scientific research that depends on the availability of human embryos can proceed with embryos no older than 14 days, this social good can proceed without paralyzing encumbrance. Yet, at the same time, the Committee does not declare that embryos of less than 14 days have no moral importance. Although it is not clear about why these early embryos deserve moral respect, it is unequivocal in declaring that they must be respected. In this way, the social problem was addressed without declaring a detailed official position on the moral status of embryos.

In a comparable manner, we have generally declined to examine the so-called "hard reasons" justifying abortion—rape, incest, or a "defective" fetus. What makes these reasons more persuasive than others? If the fetus is truly an innocent person, then surely the fact that it came into existence as a result of rape or incest is not in any possible way its fault. Or take the problem of fetuses with probable genetic or developmental abnormalities. We do not believe that killing an adolescent with Down syndrome is any less of a crime than killing another person of the same age but with 46 rather than 47 chromosomes. Why is it permissible to abort a 20 weeks' fetus with Down syndrome, but wrong to do the same to a genetically normal one?

We can take almost exactly the same questions, transforming them only to refer to newborns rather than fetuses. It is true that we now appear to have a relatively stable consensus that one should not deny life-saving therapies to a disabled infant such as one with Down syndrome when that same therapy would be given to an otherwise similar infant without the disability. Yet we do this without anything remotely like a well-founded, carefully argued social understanding about the moral worth of disabled infants and children. And there are many other social policies strongly suggesting that we do not regard the disabled, especially the mentally disabled, as possessing equal moral worth with the nondisabled. The way we often tuck them away in grievously underfunded institutions, the way we skimp on funding programs for their education and for the support of their parents—these and other policies seem to indicate a lack of moral respect for disabled persons.

At the outset, as well as at the end of life, we struggle without resolution with the idea that the quality of life a person faces ought to figure into the decisions other people make for that individual. The concept of "quality of life" is surely one of the most vague and contentious in contemporary bioethics.* Those critical of using quality of life as a factor in making treatment/nontreatment decisions see it as a convenient ideology for disposing of the defenseless and undesirable, and as a negation of the ultimate value residing in each individual person, no matter how devastated. Those in favor of considering quality of life point to the potential wastefulness of employing expensive, aggressive measures for a person whose life will not thereby be improved. Or else, some proponents argue that it is unjust to lavish resources on those with severely limited capacities for experience or accomplishment when that diminishes what will be available for those whose potential is limited principally by a shortage of resources.

There would be a stiff price to pay if we adopted clear and decisive social policies either way. If we formally denounced every vestige of quality-of-life judgments, we would be forced into untenable practices. For example, we would have to consider heart transplants for irreversibly comatose patients who were otherwise stable, since to do otherwise would be to judge that the irreversibly comatose have a lower quality of life than others, and that would be forbidden. If a heart became available

---

* See John Arras's chapter in this book for a careful analysis of the concept "quality of life."

that was compatible with such a patient, we might have to deny that tragically scarce resource to some other, fully functioning person. Or, if the resource were not limited by natural scarcity, we would be morally obliged to commit the funds to provide it for even the most devastated, where there was genuine doubt whether that was doing them any service.

If this seems unjust and wasteful, consider the alternative. An open embrace of the quality-of-life concept would mean renouncing the fundamental principle that, to paraphrase the Declaration of Independence, "All persons are created equal." It would give explicit social sanction with fatal force for drawing distinctions among admittedly innocent persons. And it would force us to declare publicly what does, and does not, impair a person's quality of life sufficiently to diminish that person's claim on society's aid. Is it physical disability? Mental disability? An IQ of 5, 25, or 50?

Formally accepting or rejecting quality-of-life criteria could result in profound social costs, both monetary and symbolic. Everyone is entitled to his own view of how we actually handle this issue in the United States, but my impression is that we permit people to make quality-of-life judgments, so long as they do not offend our moral sensibilities. When they do, we react. This, I believe, is roughly what happened in the Baby Doe (Indiana) controversy. Our notion of what acceptable quality-of-life judgments includes no longer extends to allowing Down syndrome infants to die by withholding operations that would certainly be performed on other children. Whatever the threshold of quality of life is, it is now well below Baby Doe.

The federal legislation and regulation on medical care of newborns embodied this parry-and-thrust over quality of life. After carefully worded compromise legislation was passed, the U.S. Department of Health and Human Services issued proposed regulations that explicitly denounced quality-of-life criteria (8). Despite a massive letter-writing campaign in support of DHHS's proposal, opposition from the coalition of U.S. senators who sponsored the legislation, as well as from professional organizations, forced the Department to take its denunciation of quality-of-life judgments out of the final rule. Instead, it tucked them into an appended set of "interpretive guidelines" that have no legal force (9). So the federal response was to declare that quality-of-life criteria were symbolically unacceptable, yet posed no serious barriers to those who would use them in ways that did not outrage public opinion (10).

Another effect of the Baby Doe controversy was to focus attention on the question, Whose interests may be counted in making surrogate decisions? May we count the interests of parents, siblings, nurses, physicians, or society (in the sense of its interest in preserving resources)? Or must our decisions depend solely on the infant's interests? Debate among bioethicists has uncovered ambiguities in the very idea of an infant's having certain "interests" (11), and in applying that concept, even broadly understood, to certain classes of infants, especially the neurologically devastated (12). But take a less extreme example, say a very-low-birthweight baby with multiple complications who, if she survives, will likely require care that will exhaust her parents' financial, emotional, and physical resources. Let us say these same parents already have two healthy children. Would they be justified in taking into account the interests of their other children or their own interests? How much weight, if any, could they give these considerations? These are the questions at the level of individual decisions. At the policy level we are compelled to ask what action, if any, should we take to ensure that interests other than the infant's are (or are not) taken into account. This substantive question remains unanswered. Our approach so far has been to recommend a procedural solution, the creation of Infant Bioethics Review Committees, charged generally with making decisions in accordance with the infant's well-being, rather than trying to extensively specify what counts as well-being, and whether it includes the interests of other family members.

The Problem of Justice

Not all difficult social policy decisions involve stark value conflicts, either manifest or latent. Some of the toughest involve choices among desirable options. Societies must decide what worthwhile practices they will support, and how generously. Once a technology such as artificial insemination from a donor (AID) or *in vitro* fertilization works well enough to be deemed practical, and if there are no strenuous moral objections to it, we must still choose whether or not to support it with public funds or take other measures to ensure its widespread availability. The Warnock Committee mentioned earlier did indeed recommend that these two methods for overcoming infertility be available within Britain's National Health Service (13). For the most part, in the United States these services are available only to those who can pay for them. The different choices in the two countries bespeak quite different judgments about the place of infertility therapies in a system of just health care. The contrast is all the more pointed when we realize that Britain spends only about one-half as much of their gross national product on health care as does the United States (14).

Deciding that a procedure is ethically sound is merely a necessary condition for the quite separate questions whether we should facilitate people's efforts to obtain it, or whether we should actually provide it at public expense. There are any number of good things in life that are left to individuals to obtain for themselves. Normally, health care has been much more likely than most other goods to be provided for collectively, by insurance, by government funding, or by charity. The debate over whether to fund AID and IVF will turn, most likely, on arguments about whether they are like other kinds of health care, that is, therapies intended to cure diseases or alleviate suffering, or whether they are another sort of social service, doing good for people, but not deserving the same kind of public financial support as "genuine" health care.

Deciding whether to provide infertility therapies, while it will involve questions about the nature of health and disease, is also a problem of justice. To a considerable extent, the debate over whether infertility is a disease is an argument over whether to count it as a "natural" injustice, since in general diseases are seen as naturally caused differences among individuals that are not their fault, and that place people at an undeserved disadvantage. Labeling something a "disease," then, characterizes it as a condition appropriate for socially supported amelioration, an injustice society ought to consider remediating (15).

Once something is identified as a candidate for remediation, there are still values to be considered. Given finite resources, how do these victims of "natural" injustice stack up against other victims? Who is more deserving? What are the respective costs for helping one group as opposed to another? In this way, complex ideas about justice, including notions of desert and choice, interact with concerns about efficiency to affect our perception of what a reasonable set of policies would be.

Social Policy and the Notion of 'Maternal Responsibility'

The time has come to apply what has been said to a set of issues. Any of a large number could be chosen, but let us look at a group centering on the concept of maternal responsibility. The key factual premise is that the behavior of the mother, both before and during pregnancy, can affect the health of the child that the embryo and later the fetus will become. We can leave aside for now the problem of the moral status of the unwanted embryo and fetus, and focus exclusively on those who are intended to be carried to term.

The first moral point is that the timing of a harm done to a person is not of itself relevant to our moral judgment about the wrongness of the act causing the harm, or to the blameworthiness of the agent (or agents) of harm. People tend to be confused about this, particularly when the point is applied to our responsibilities to a fetus or embryo, because of several other factors that are also relevant to judgments about the morality of acts that might harm the child-to-be. For example, the things we might do to harm a fetus or embryo are usually complex acts affecting the mother as well as possibly several other people. These acts usually carry with them only a small probability of harm, and the harms are typically multiply determined, so it is difficult even in retrospect to assign causation unequivocally. (What caused the slight neurological damage to the baby? Was it that bottle of wine the mother shared in? Was it her work in the pigment division of the paint factory? Was it the polluted air of her city?) My point is simply that we can and should use the same criteria for judging the morality of acts (or policies) with potential for harming embryos or fetuses who are destined to become children as we would use to judge any other sort of act (or policy).

It is crucial to see that this point about morality and children-to-be *does not* mean that only pregnant women have responsibilities toward them, nor does it require that women sacrifice all other responsibilities or claims they might have to the welfare of their fetuses or embryos. And, above all for the subject of this chapter, it does not mean that society should step in to enforce the child-to-be's claims against the mother or anyone else, or permit others to make policies doing the same.

To illuminate these points, I will skip over the more common issues such as whether and how to encourage mothers to avoid harming their fetuses by excessive drinking or by smoking. Because of the great number of women and children-to-be affected, these are important questions. But two other problems more clearly illuminate the issues: so-called fetal protection policies imposed by corporations, and mothers with phenylketonuria, whose fetuses are at grave risk of harm.

Fetal protection policies, formal and informal, have been in effect in an unknown but in all probability a large number of industrial corporations. Many chemicals and types of radiation are known or believed to be harmful to developing fetuses, and companies have often responded to these threats with policies that remove women from work sites where exposures are possible. They may accomplish this by refusing to hire "potentially pregnant" women (which in many instances means all women roughly between 15 and 50 who are not certifiably sterile), by transferring them, or by firing them (16).

A number of ethical questions can be raised about these fetal protection policies, and I have discussed some of them elsewhere (17). Here I want to concentrate on how I believe we ought to think about a parent's responsibility for his or her child-to-be, when employment may carry risk. The first point is that the mother may not be the only source of risk. While the scientific evidence is by no means conclusive, it does suggest that occupational harms may also be transmitted through fathers (18). And, of course, the fetus may be exposed to chemicals or radiation from environmental, nonoccupational sources.

A second consideration relies on the scientific evidence suggesting that all or most occupational exposures likely to be risky to fetuses are also likely to cause harm to adult workers. At the chromosomal level, the mechanisms of fetal toxicity are similar or identical to the mechanisms of carcinogenesis and mutagenesis (19). Exposures low enough to be tolerable risks to adult workers are also likely to pose a low probability of harm to fetuses. The question then amounts to whether a parent is justified in exposing his or her child-to-be to a low-probability risk of a harm of unknown magnitude (depending of the particulars, anywhere from undetectable minor damage to severe, lifelong devastation).

Our answers to such questions are often conditioned by our beliefs about mother-child relationships, our attitudes about working mothers, and our notions about the fetus. It would be helpful to find a comparable case that preserved the central moral features of this one, without the excess baggage of the mother-fetus connection. For one thing, we can note that whatever our moral duties are to a fetus, they can equal but not exceed our duties to our born children. The child then, constitutes an upper bound for duties to the fetus or embryo. If exposing our children to particular risks was judged morally acceptable, then exposing a fetus or embryo to a comparable risk must also be acceptable.

Take an example of a father who is offered a job in a community rich in petrochemical plants. The job would offer much better pay, benefits, and schools than his current work in a rural town. But moving his wife and children to the new city would mean exposing them to plant emissions and the low but nonetheless increased risk of cancer those emissions pose. Would that man be justified in making an all-things-considered decision to accept those increased risks to his family's health in order to gain the other goods the new job makes possible? We might disagree with the man's decision to take the job, but we would not say that his choice was immoral. In precisely the same way, we would not judge as immoral a woman's choice to work under conditions of comparable risk to her fetus and comparable benefit to her fetus, herself, and the remainder of her family.

Under these circumstances, corporate policies that denied jobs to women could not be justified on the grounds that they "protected" fetuses against the ignorant or immoral decisions of their prospective mothers. For one thing, our hypothetical case shows that decisions to work under conditions of some degree of risk to a fetus (or child) may be morally defensible. We may regret that people are faced with such a Hobson's choice, and strive to create a society where parents do not have to choose between risking their own, or their children's—born and unborn—health. But we cannot justify policies stripping only prospective mothers of such choices, when in so doing we reduce even further the already limited employment opportunities many women face.

If the facts were different, if we knew of an "occupational thalidomide"—a substance devastating to fetuses or embryos yet utterly harmless to adults at the same exposures—then we might come to a different conclusion. We would be forced to weigh more carefully the costs to women's employment opportunities and the risks to fetal health against the increased production costs to industry and the higher market price of the goods produced if we chose to require stricter exposure controls. But, we probably do not face such a choice yet, at least not in the occupational theater. There is one area, though, where the facts of fetal risk are so firmly and tragically established that we do confront a need to make some difficult social policy choices. This is the problem of mothers with the inherited metabolic abnormality phenylketonuria, commonly known as PKU.

Thanks to the development of a test to detect PKU in newborns and a special diet to control the intake of the amino acid phenylalanine, hundreds of people have been spared the ravages of unmanaged PKU. Infants with PKU are unable to metabolize phenylalanine properly. Consequently, their developing brains are bathed in toxic concentrations of phenylalanine and its metabolites. The result is usually severe retardation and hyperactivity. For over 20 years now in the United States, babies have been routinely tested for PKU. Once they are identified, they are placed on a diet that strictly limits the amount of phenylalanine they receive. Bland, boring, and expensive, the diet is frequently abandoned sometime during or shortly after adolescence. Though the evidence is far from complete, it appears that once the brain has completed its development, it is not so susceptible to damage from PKU.

We now have a generation of young men and women with PKU who lead essentially normal lives, who can work, love, and have children of their own. Here is where the problem arises. What does the damage to the developing brain is not the defective gene itself, but the high levels of phenylalanine and its metabolites in the bloodstream. If a woman with PKU becomes pregnant while on a normal diet, dangerously high levels of these substances will be in her blood and will pass through the placenta to attack the brain of her fetus. This will be true even if, as is almost certain, the fetus itself does not have the genetic abnormality associated with PKU.

The scientific evidence linking maternal PKU with developmental disorders in offspring is firm and tragic. A study of 444 births to mothers with PKU found a strong dose-response relationship between maternal blood levels of PKU and neurological damage to the child (20). Roughly two-thirds of the mothers had PKU levels over 20. Ninety-two percent of their infants were retarded, and 73 percent were microcephalic. About one-ninth of the mothers had PKU levels of between 3 and 10. Twenty-one percent of their children were retarded, 24 percent microcephalic. (These figures contrast with non-PKU mothers, 5 percent of whose children will be retarded, and 4.8 percent microcephalic.)

We have good reason to believe, then, that a woman with PKU who does not observe the low-phenylalanine diet places her child-to-be at a very high risk, approaching certainty, of severe harm. (The contrast with the choice faced by women in potentially toxic, but very-low-probability situations should be obvious.) At the level of the practice, do women with PKU have a moral responsibility to follow the low-phenylalanine diet when they are planning to become pregnant? At the policy level, what social policies should we adopt to minimize the likelihood of neurologically devastated children being born to mothers with PKU?

The first question is clearly about individual moral responsibility. It is worth discussing briefly here. Several factors seem relevant. First, the potential harm to the child-to-be is grievous and highly probable. Second, it appears to be quite avoidable. Third, no one else is in position to protect the fetus other than the mother. Fourth, what a mother with PKU would need to do to protect her fetus is unpleasant, perhaps (the dull diet), but temporary, and not threatening to any of her vital interests. It seems then that a woman with PKU does have a moral obligation to avoid harming her child-to-be by adhering to the special diet if she intends to become pregnant, and if she intends to bear that fetus to term.

If we find a social consensus that women with PKU have such moral responsibilities, what if anything follows about social policy? As I said earlier, a clear judgment about the morality (or immorality) of particular acts or practices is neither a necessary nor a sufficient condition for establishing social policy. It will count as one among many factors, some directly relevant to ethics, others not so related.

In this particular case, we have many choices. We could ignore it. We could try to educate women with PKU about the danger to their children, relying on the benign intentions parents typically show their offspring. This educational effort could be relatively passive, waiting for the women to come for help, or it could be aggressive, reaching out to them.

But we are not limited to such noncoercive options, at least not by logic alone. We could try to prevent pregnancies among PKU women by requiring them to use contraceptives, or for that matter by enforced sterilization. We could monitor their diets during pregnancy, and perhaps incarcerate them if they deviated from it. Of course, we are not doing any of these coercive things for a variety of reasons, some moral, some pragmatic. Forced contraception is morally abhorent and is difficult to accomplish as well. Forcible sterilization might be more achievable but even more ethically reprehensible than coercive contraception. Monitoring diet would be well-nigh impossible, and incarceration a drastic infringement of personal liberty that we should undertake only with compelling evidence of wrongdoing.

In fact, the policy we now pursue is the positive one of aggressive education with outreach. Does this mean that some pregnancies will escape the net? Unfortunately, it probably does, although we hope and expect that the number will be very small. Is that an acceptable price to pay for a policy that tries hard to respect the dignity and liberty of women with PKU? This is indeed a moral question, a question about the morality of a particular social policy.

Some Comments about Ethics and Social Policy

As societies struggle to craft sensible and morally defensible policies for problems at the outset of life, there are some evils to be avoided. On the one hand, there are often temptations to adopt *moralistic* policies. By this I mean policies shaped according to a narrow conception of the values appropriate to policymaking, specifically, a narrow set of moral concerns. This amounts to ignoring a wide range of other values, moral and nonmoral, that are relevant and significant. The price a society pays for moralistic policymaking includes widespread disobedience, disrespect, and disaffection, as well as a suspicion that ethics should have no role in social policy.

This suspicion of ethics in policy easily leads to the other extreme, amoral policymaking in the style of realpolitik. Claiming that ethics can and should have nothing to do with policy, this view has at least two fatal flaws. First, it robs the deliberative cycle of considering, establishing, critiquing, and revising policies of the powerful corrective force of moral criticism. It is important to be able to say if a policy is unfair, unjust, unnecessarily restrictive of personal liberty, or otherwise ethically dubious. Second, the amoral approach fails to appreciate that, in a democracy at least, policies ultimately rest on a social consensus that they are acceptable, including the conviction that they are *morally* acceptable. Failure to be attentive to the moral dimensions of policies at the outset of life could undermine those very policies.

A last concern is what happens when societies adopt policies offensive to the moral convictions of some individuals. At this time in the United States, whatever policy is adopted toward abortion will be morally offensive to some. If abortion is tolerated, those who believe it is murder are outraged; if abortion is banned or severely restricted, those who believe this is a serious infringement on the rights of women will feel the same.

Two things may be said about this. First, the distinction between tolerating and forcing becomes highly salient in these dilemmas. I suspect there would be a public outcry if the state ever got into the business of compelling abortions for whatever reason. In the face of profound disagreement, societies prefer to tolerate differences in beliefs and behaviors, rather than enforce one particular view. This does mean that certain evils may be permitted, but that is generally preferable to having the state enforce one particular view of morality on a dissenting majority.

Whether the state tolerates differences or enforces one view, individuals may believe that wrongs, even grave wrongs, are being done. (It makes a great deal of difference whether those wrongs are being compelled by or done at the behest of the state, or the state remains neutral, tolerating, but not forcing.) Civil disobedience, in the sense of refusing to comply with state decrees, has long been an honorable option for citizens who believe that the state commands a moral wrong. There is considerable literature on the topic (21). The situation is somewhat different when the state tolerates but does not command. This is the issue faced by those in the United States today who believe that abortion is plainly murder. They have been fairly successful in extirpating state support for abortion (though this effort itself raises a number of questions about fairness, when, for example, federal funding for abortions for the poor is withdrawn, leaving poor women with the right, but not the means, to procure abortions). But they must still decide what to do with respect to those abortions that are tolerated. It is important to see here that the resort to violence is *not* the same sort of civil disobedience as refusal to comply with what one believes is an immoral state decree. It is action of another, distinctive kind and requires a different sort of moral justification. Whether it should be justified or condemned is a moral problem in social and political philosophy, one likely to remain with us for some time.

References

1. Barbara Cohen, "Surrogate Mothers: Whose Baby Is It?," *American Journal of Law and Medicine 10*, no. 3 (1984): 243–85.
2. *Griswold v. State of Connecticut,* Supreme Court of the United States, 1965, 381 U.S. 479, 85 s.Ct. 1678, 14 L.Ed.2d 510. The excerpt quoted was from the majority opinion delivered by Justice Douglas.
3. A summary of much of the research bearing on these issues is available in Peter Budetti, Nancy Barrand, Peggy McManus, and LuAnn Heinen, "The Costs and Effectiveness of Neonatal Intensive Care," Case Study 10 on *The Implications of Cost-Effectiveness Analysis of Medical Technology,* a series of background papers commissioned by the U.S. Congress Office of Technology Assessment. It is available from the Government Printing Office as OTY-BP-H-9(10), August, 1981.
4. Kristin Luker, *Abortion and the Politics of Motherhood* (Berkeley: University of California Press, 1984).
5. U.S. Senate, Senate Judiciary Committee, Subcommittee on Constitutional Amendments. *Hearings to Consider S.J. Res. 119 and S.J. Res. 130.*
6. Report of the Committee of Inquiry into Human Fertilisation and Embryology, United Kingdom Department of Health and Social Security (London: HMSO, July 1984). This Committee was chaired by dame Mary Warnock, a British philosopher, and has come to be known as the Warnock Committee.
7. Ibid. The phrases quoted may be found on pp. 63 and 64 of the text, and as recommendations 42 and 43 on p. 84.
8. U.S. Department of Health and Human Services, 45 CFR Part 1340 "Child Abuse and Neglect Prevention and Treatment Program: Notice of Proposed Rulemaking," *Federal Register 49,* 238 (Dec. 10, 1984).
9. U.S. Department of Health and Human Services, 45 CFR Part 1340 "Child Abuse and Neglect Prevention and Treatment Program: Final Rule" and "Model Guidelines for Health Care Providers to Establish Infant Care Review Committees: Notice," *Federal Register 50,* 72 (April 15, 1985).
10. Thomas H. Murray, "The Final, Anticlimactic Rule on Baby Doe," *Hastings Center Report* (June 1985): 5–9.
11. Martin Benjamin, "The Newborn's Interest In Continued Life: A Sentimental Fiction," *Bioethics Reporter 1* (1983): 5–7.
12. John D. Arras, "Toward an Ethic of Ambiguity," *Hastings Center Report* (April 1984): 25–33.
13. The Warnock Committee's support for IVF is explicit in recommendation 40 (p. 84 of the Report of the Committee). Their support for AID (and AIH) may be deduced from their general comments in chapter 4 of the Report (pp. 17–28).
14. Henry J. Aaron and William B. Schwartz, *The Painful Prescription: Rationing Hospital Care* (Washington, D.C.: Brookings Institution, 1984).
15. There is much more to be said about disease, its relation to need and justification of public provision of health services, etc. Normal Daniels' comments in "Health Care Needs and Distributive Justice," in Ronald Bayer, Arthur L. Caplan, and Norman Daniels, eds., *In Search of Equity: Health Needs and the Health Care System* (New York: Plenum Press, 1983) are a useful starting point.

ETHICS AND SOCIAL POLICY

16. U.S. Congress Office of Technology Assessment, *Reproductive Hazards in the Workplace* (Washington, D.C.: Government Printing Office, Dec. 1985).

17. Thomas H. Murray, "Who Do Fetal Protection Policies Really Protect?," *Technology Review* (Oct. 1985): 12–13.

18. U.S. Congress Office of Technology Assessment, *Reproductive Hazards in the Workplace;* see especially the chapter "Evidence for Workplace Hazards to Reproductive Function."

19. J. J. Yunis, "The Chromosomal Basis of Human Neoplasia," *Science 221* (July 15, 1983): 227–36. See also J. B. Ward, Jr., "Issues in Monitoring Population Exposures," in H. F. Stitch, ed., *Carcinogens and Mutagens in the Environment: Volume IV: The Workplace* (Boca Raton, Fla.: CRC Press, 1985).

20. H. L. Levy et al., "Effects of Untreated Maternal PKU and Hyperphenylalanemia on the Fetus," *New England Journal of Medicine 309*, 21 (Nov. 24, 1983): 1269–74.

21. Perhaps the best known source on civil disobedience is Henry David Thoreau's essay by the same name. For a more recent discussion, see Michael Walzer, *Obligations: Essays on Disobedience, War, and Citizenship* (New York: Simon and Schuster (Clarion), 1971).

Index

Index